Workbook and Lab Manual for Mosby's Pharmacy Technician: Principles and Practice

3rd edition

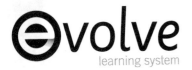
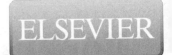
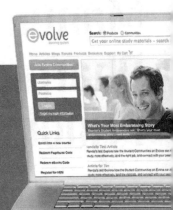

Workbook and Lab Manual for Mosby's Pharmacy Technician: Principles and Practice

3rd edition

Teresa Hopper, BS, CPhT
Instructor of Pharmacy Technology
Boston Reed College
Napa, California

Workbook Material Provided by:
Shelby L. Newberry, MCPhT
Pharmacy Technician Program Director
Vatterott College of Kansas City
Kansas City, Missouri

Additional Material Provided by:
Bobbi Steelman, CPhT
Program Leader of Pharmacy Technology Program
Pharmacy Technician Program Manager
Daymar College
Bowling Green, Kentucky

ELSEVIER
SAUNDERS

ELSEVIER
SAUNDERS

3251 Riverport Lane
St. Louis, Missouri 63043

WORKBOOK AND LAB MANUAL FOR MOSBY'S
PHARMACY TECHNICIAN

ISBN: 978-1-4377-0671-0

Notices

Knowledge and best practice in this field are constantly changing. As new research and experience broaden our understanding, changes in research methods, professional practices, or medical treatment may become necessary.

Practitioners and researchers must always rely on their own experience and knowledge in evaluating and using any information, methods, compounds, or experiments described herein. In using such information or methods they should be mindful of their own safety and the safety of others, including parties for whom they have a professional responsibility.

With respect to any drug or pharmaceutical products identified, readers are advised to check the most current information provided (i) on procedures featured or (ii) by the manufacturer of each product to be administered, to verify the recommended dose or formula, the method and duration of administration, and contraindications. It is the responsibility of practitioners, relying on their own experience and knowledge of their patients, to make diagnoses, to determine dosages and the best treatment for each individual patient, and to take all appropriate safety precautions.

To the fullest extent of the law, neither the Publisher nor the authors, contributors, or editors, assume any liability for any injury and/or damage to persons or property as a matter of products liability, negligence or otherwise, or from any use or operation of any methods, products, instructions, or ideas contained in the material herein.

Previous editions copyrighted 2007, 2004

Publishing Director: Andrew Allen
Senior Acquisitions Editor: Jennifer Janson
Developmental Editor: Kelly Brinkman
Publishing Services Manager: Julie Eddy
Senior Project Manager: Rich Barber

Printed in the United States

Last digit is the print number: 9   8   7   6   5   4   3

Preface

This student workbook and lab manual is designed to help you master the information and skills presented in your textbook: *Mosby's Pharmacy Technician: Principles and Practice*, 3rd edition. The various types of exercises will challenge your knowledge, help further reinforce key content, allow you to gauge your understanding of the subject matter, and demonstrate important concepts in the lab setting. This combination workbook and lab manual is divided into three separate areas for each chapter in the textbook: Reinforce Key Concepts, Reflect Critically, and Relate to Practice. Each of these three sections focus on activities for students that will maximize their understanding of the content taught in the book.

The types of activities available in this workbook and lab manual are listed and described below:

REINFORCE KEY CONCEPTS

- *Terms and Definitions:* Terms and definitions are listed, preceded by a letter. You are to read each statement following the list, and write in the letter that represents the correct response. This exercise helps you recall the many terms that are introduced to you in each chapter. Your textbook conveniently lists this information at the beginning of each chapter. If you find you are not sure of any of your responses, you can easily turn to the appropriate chapter to refresh your memory.
- *Fill in the Blanks:* Complete each statement by filling in the blanks. This exercise gives you the opportunity to specifically apply the vocabulary you have learned within the context of pharmacy.
- *True or False:* Test your knowledge of the validity of the statements. If you think a statement is true, write a "T" in the blank preceding the statement; if you believe it is a false statement, write in an "F." Completing these exercises helps you immediately to recognize content of which you are unsure. You can then review and strengthen your understanding of the material by rereading that particular section in your textbook.
- *Multiple Choice:* You are to select the one best answer to complete the numbered questions by circling the letter preceding the answer you have selected. This is the type of question in which your first response is usually the correct reply. If you are not sure, then you can easily review the subject in question.
- *System Identifier:* Each chapter devoted to a body system features an illustration of the system with its organs numbered. You are asked to identify the organs contained in the body system. This visual exercise helps further reinforce your knowledge of anatomy. Questions in these chapters test you on the anatomy and physiology of the system, diseases and conditions that may occur within this system, and the medications prescribed to treat such illnesses.
- *Matching:* These exercises provide you with essential practice in matching controlled substance drug schedules with given drug names. Ease of recognition is essential in your chosen profession. If you are not sure of some of your responses, you can then refer back to your textbook for further study.
- *Conversion and Calculation:* These questions require you to convert measurements, thereby applying what you have learned.
- *Research Activities:* You are asked to use the Internet as a research tool to assist you in locating essential information. Featured websites address such topics as the scope of practice for pharmacy technicians and where to find information on controlled substances and recalls.

REFLECT CRITICALLY

- *Critical Thinking:* This exercise tests your accumulated knowledge of each chapter by giving you scenarios to solve. You are asked to draw upon your knowledge of pharmacy and direct it to specific situations. This is a good test of your understanding of key concepts. If any of these questions stump you, refer back to your textbook for further study, or ask your instructor for clarification.

RELATE TO PRACTICE

- *Lab Activities:* Labs for each chapter will help you master such skills as gram staining, inventory management, compounding, and aseptic technique. These labs offer you many opportunities for hands-on reinforcements of what you have learned in your textbook.

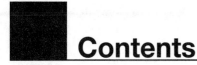

Contents

Workbook and Lab Manual for Mosby's Pharmacy Technician: Principles and Practice

3rd edition

1 History of Medicine and Pharmacy

REINFORCE KEY CONCEPTS

TERMS AND DEFINITIONS

Select the correct term from the following list and write the corresponding letter in the blank next to the statement.

A. Apothecary
B. Bloodletting
C. Inpatient pharmacy
D. Medicine
E. Leeches
F. Staff of Asclepius
G. Caduceus
H. Shaman
I. Protocol
J. Laudanum

_____ 1. The practice of draining blood thought to release illness

_____ 2. The science and art of dealing with the maintenance of health

_____ 3. Segmented worm that attaches to the skin

_____ 4. Symbol of the medical profession

_____ 5. Latin term for pharmacist

_____ 6. A pharmacy in a hospital or institutional setting

_____ 7. A spiritual person in a tribe who cares for the spiritual, medicinal, and physical health of the tribe

_____ 8. Often confused as the symbol of the medical field

_____ 9. Set of standards written by a hospital or insurance company for patient treatment

_____ 10. A mixture of opium and alcohol used through the 1800s

IMPORTANT PEOPLE WHO HAVE INFLUENCED THE HISTORY OF MEDICINE

Select the correct name from the following list and write the corresponding letter in the blank next to the description.

A. Aristotle
B. Asclepius
C. Galen
D. Hippocrates
E. Roger Bacon
F. Gregor Mendel
G. Paracelsus

_____ 1. Scientist and monk, known as the father of genetics

_____ 2. Considered god of healing and medicine

_____ 3. Greek philosopher and scientist

_____ 4. Greek philosopher and physician, considered the father of medicine

_____ 5. English scientist responsible for scientific methods

_____ 6. Greek physician who proved that blood flowed through arteries

_____ 7. Swiss physician, philosopher, and scientist

1

MULTIPLE CHOICE

Complete each question by circling the best answer.

1. The placebo effect:
   A. Works from the outside of the body to the inside
   B. Works by placing the drug over the area to be treated
   C. Works because the patient strongly believes it will work
   D. Works only after midnight

2. Trephining is:
   A. A radical treatment that lasted for hundreds of years
   B. A term used to describe menstrual bleeding
   C. Draining of poisonous blood from the sick person
   D. An incision into the skull to create an exit portal for disease

3. In early America, physicians were:
   A. Responsible for diagnosing conditions
   B. Responsible for preparing the necessary remedy
   C. The first druggists
   D. All of the above

4. The division between physicians and pharmacists began after the:
   A. Korean War
   B. Civil War
   C. Vietnam War
   D. Cold War

5. Alexander Fleming:
   A. Studied medicine from a shaman
   B. Opened the first pharmacy in America
   C. Discovered penicillin
   D. Created the Caduceus

6. Early remedies in American history included:
   A. Cinchona bark (quinine) to treat malaria
   B. Mercury to treat syphilis
   C. Opium and alcohol to treat pain
   D. All of the above

7. The first pharmacy technicians were:
   A. Military personnel
   B. High school graduates
   C. Family members of the pharmacist
   D. Certified pharmacy technicians (CPhTs)

8. Archeological discoveries have unearthed civilizations that documented:
    A. The use of penicillin in Egypt
    B. The use of minerals, animals, and plants to heal the sick
    C. The first pharmacists
    D. The first written prescription

9. In some states, today's typical pharmacy technician:
    A. Is required to do an array of tasks
    B. Is required to be educated and receive on-the-job training
    C. Is a family member of the pharmacist
    D. Both A and B

10. How can technicians gain the trust of the patients they serve?
    A. Education
    B. Training
    C. Good communication skills
    D. All of the above

11. The concept that doctors act only for the good of the patient and keep confidential what they learn about their patients reflects the:
    A. Galenic oath
    B. Corpus Hippocratum
    C. Hippocratic oath
    D. De Materia Medica

12. The effectiveness of the opium and alcohol mixture known as Laudanum was surpassed only by its:
    A. Addictiveness
    B. Availability
    C. Adverse effects
    D. All of the above

13. Some of the instruments used earliest for bloodletting were:
    A. Thorns
    B. Sharp bones
    C. Shark teeth
    D. All of the above

14. The first synthetic drug, a(n) _____, was discovered by Gerhard Domagk.
    A. Opioid
    B. Benzodiazepine
    C. Sulfonamide
    D. Cephalosporin

15. Some physicians are not eager to have pharmacists:
    A. Writing medication orders
    B. Administering shots
    C. Diagnosing patients
    D. Making more money than physicians

FILL IN THE BLANK

Answer each question by completing the statement in the space provided.

1. Technicians help pharmacists by preparing _____ and _____.

2. Name four duties of pharmacy technicians in a hospital setting:

   A. _____

   B. _____

   C. _____

   D. _____

3. Name two areas of pharmacy in which a pharmacist can specialize:

   A. _____

   B. _____

4. The most important quality a technician can develop when working with patients is _____.

5. Each year, more pharmacy employers are requiring a certain level of _____ from their technicians.

SHORT ANSWER

Write a short response to each question in the space provided.

1. State the first line of the Hippocratic oath.

   _____

   _____

2. What is the difference between an opioid and opium?

   _____

   _____

   _____

3. What does the term *dogma* mean?

   _____

   _____

4. What must a technician do to gain the trust of the patient?

   _____

   _____

5. What duties do today's pharmacy technician perform that once were included as duties of the traditional pharmacist?

   _____

   _____

RESEARCH ACTIVITY

Follow the instructions given in each exercise and provide a response.

1. Access the website *www.ptcb.org* and investigate the duties outlined for pharmacy technicians.

2. Access the website *www.pharmacy.wsu.edu/history*. List five facts from the account of the history of pharmacy.

REFLECT CRITICALLY

CRITICAL THINKING

Reply to each question based on what you have learned in the chapter.

1. One of the most important aspects of a pharmacy technician's job is to gain the trust of the pharmacist. How would you, as a new technician on the job, go about gaining the trust of the pharmacist?

2. What changes have you observed in pharmacy as a consumer over the years?

3. How have medicinal treatments changed from ancient beliefs to present-day practices? Start with the shamans and conclude with twenty-first century medicine.

3 Pharmacy Ethics, Competencies, Associations, and Settings for Technicians

TRUE OR FALSE

Write T or F next to each statement.

___T___ 1. Each of the 50 states in the United States has standardized the qualifications and job descriptions for pharmacy technicians.

___T___ 2. Each state has its own board of pharmacy that is overseen by the NABP.

___F___ 3. Pharmacy technicians perform nondiscretionary tasks, such as counseling patients.

___T___ 4. *Inpatient pharmacy* refers to pharmacy for patients who are in the hospital for an overnight stay or longer.

___F___ 5. Running an outpatient pharmacy is one of the most difficult tasks in pharmacy.

___F___ 6. Knowledge of pharmacy law is not essential to work in a pharmacy environment.

___F___ 7. Typing speed required by most pharmacy employers is at least 15 WPM.

___T___ 8. Pharmacy technicians are taking over many of the traditional roles of the pharmacist.

___F___ 9. The term *communication skill* refers to verbal skills only.

___T___ 10. Allowing patients to express their frustrations, being a good listener, and doing one's best to help people are what being a professional is all about.

PHARMACY TECHNICIAN JOB OPPORTUNITIES

Select the correct job from the following list and write the corresponding letter in the blank next to the description.

A. Inventory technician
B. Robot filler
C. Chemo technician
D. Clinical technician
E. Insurance technician
F. Technician recruiter
G. Technician trainer
H. Pharmacy business management operator
I. Computer support technician
J. Poison control call center operator

___G___ 1. Trains newly hired technicians in computer programs and other skills relevant to the pharmacy

___C___ 2. Receives orders and prepares all chemotherapeutic agents

___B___ 3. Supports personnel by helping with automated medication dispensing systems

___E___ 4. Knows the guidelines of Medicare, Blue Cross, and other insurance companies

___F___ 5. Recruits technicians into outpatient or temporary agencies

___A___ 6. Orders and bills all stock

___J___ 7. Screens incoming calls and transfers calls to 911 operator or pharmacist; authorized to take the call if it concerns a minor issue

___D___ 8. Assists the pharmacist with tracking patients' medications or compiling data for drug utilization study

___I___ 9. Is trained to load mechanical dispensing equipment and keep it running smoothly

___H___ 10. Hires technicians to help customers over the phone

TERMS AND DEFINITIONS

Select the correct term from the following list and write the corresponding letter in the blank next to the statement.

A. Communication
B. American Association of
   Pharmacy Technicians
C. Confidentiality
D. Morals
E. Ethics
F. American Society of Health-System
   Pharmacists
G. Professionalism
H. National Pharmacy Technician
   Association

___C___ 1. Keeping privileged information about a customer from being disclosed without the person's consent

___H___ 2. Primarily for pharmacy technicians, founded in 1999

___A___ 3. The ability to express oneself in a way that is readily and clearly understood

___D___ 4. Ethics, honorable beliefs

___E___ 5. The values and morals used within a profession

___B___ 6. First pharmacy technician association formed in 1979, run by volunteer technicians

___G___ 7. Conforming to right principles of conduct (work ethics) as accepted by others in the profession

___F___ 8. Focuses on quality standards of pharmaceutical services and education in health systems

MULTIPLE CHOICE

Complete each question by circling the best answer:

1. The board of pharmacy:
   A. Registers pharmacists and technicians
   B. Provides a way for consumers to report complaints, problems, or illegal pharmacy actions
   C. Reviews and updates current pharmacy rules and regulations
   D. All of the above

2. The term *nondiscretionary* means that technicians can perform:
   A. Tasks that require little or no thought
   B. Tasks in a pharmacy setting that must be checked and approved by a pharmacist
   C. Tasks that require interpretation of scientific studies
   D. Tasks that are unethical

3. The National Certification Examination for Pharmacy Technicians is given:
   A. 50 times a year
   B. Four times a year
   C. Daily by appointment only
   D. Three times a year

4. Which of the following is *not* a goal of the Pharmacy Technician Certification Board?
   A. To ensure that technicians work equally and for the same pay as pharmacists
   B. To provide improved patient care and service
   C. To create a minimum standard of knowledge
   D. To help employers determine the technician's knowledge base

5. Which of the following is *not* an eligibility requirement for taking the PTCB exam?
   A. High school diploma
   B. Graduate of a pharmacy technician program
   C. No convictions for a drug-related felony
   D. GED

6. What factors must be considered before a person can be a competent pharmacy technician?
   A. Job duties
   B. Communication skills
   C. Ethics
   D. All of the above

7. Which of the following is considered a way of communicating?
   A. Speaking
   B. Listening
   C. Body language
   D. All of the above

8. Which of the following is *not* considered professional in appearance?
   A. Wedding ring
   B. Earring
   C. Nose ring
   D. Engagement ring

9. Working ethically is:
   A. Doing what is right for your beliefs
   B. Doing what is right for the patient
   C. Giving the patient everything he/she wants
   D. Showing up for work on time every day

10. Pharmacy technicians have access to confidential patient information, such as:
    A. Medical conditions
    B. Vehicle identification number
    C. Driver's license number
    D. All of the above

FILL IN THE BLANK

Answer each question by completing the statement in the space provided.

1. _____ and _____ help pharmacy management more easily choose the most competent technician to fill the position.

2. A _____ is a job, occupation, or line of work that becomes a career through obtaining specialized knowledge.

3. Certified technicians use the designation _____ after their name.

4. _____ hours of CE are required yearly to retain certification as a certified pharmacy technician.

5. Pharmacy protocol usually outlines what is _____ and _____ with regard to appearance.

6. What types of pharmacy knowledge are tested in the PTCB certification exam?

   A. _____

   B. _____

   C. _____

   D. _____

   E. _____

7. Special consideration should be given to those patients who are _____ _____.

8. Many people make an instant judgment of others within the _____ _____ _____ of meeting.

9. Pharmacies use _____ daily; _____ must be developed for pharmacy personnel.

10. Attaining increased _____ _____, including becoming _____ _____ _____, opens more doors for technicians in pharmacy.

RESEARCH ACTIVITIES

Follow the instructions given in each exercise and provide a response.

1. Call or visit a local retail or hospital pharmacy. Ask the lead technician or the pharmacist in charge the following questions:

   A. What qualifications do you require for technicians in your pharmacy?

   B. What duties do your technicians perform?

   C. Do you require certification?

2. Access the website *http://pharmacytechnician.org*. Read what this organization is doing for pharmacy technicians and find out about the requirements for membership.

3. What types of activities or benefits do the ASHP and the APhA offer technicians?

REFLECT CRITICALLY

CRITICAL THINKING

Reply to each question based on what you have learned in the chapter.

1. You have been asked to advise someone interested in becoming a pharmacy technician. How would you advise this person?

   I would recommend you look online at available classes to get certified and research online too what the job entails and what kind of tech you wish to be. Inpatient vs outpatient vs in-home? what is your background and do you have math skills?

2. What is your definition of professionalism with regard to pharmacy technicians?

   Professionalism is maintaining a conservative, dignified and un-assuming look. It is behaving in a calm and collected way and not being ostentatious or overly loud. It is also about respecting your fellow co-worker and patient.

3. How long do you think new pharmacy technicians should receive training when starting a new job?

   New techs should be trained on a sliding scale depending on how complex the job is. Maybe a month or two is sufficient at first to learn all the basics and acquire some job confidence.

4. What does your state Practice Act require of pharmacy technicians?

   Requires 120 hours of Pharm tech training at a classroom, a high school diploma, no drug-related felonies, and certification by the PTCB. Also externships at a pharm tech site.

5. What do you know about the pharmacy technician's scope of practice in your state?

   The scope is huge, with many different opportunities. Can work inpatient, outpatient, at an assisted living facility, in someone's home, over the phone, or at a laboratory. There are an overwhelming amount of possibilities.

LAB SCENARIOS

Interviewing for a Pharmacy Technician Position

Objective: To prepare a pharmacy technician student for a pharmacy technician interview.

After completing your pharmacy technician program, you are ready to find your first position as a pharmacy technician. This can be a very exciting time in your life. It is extremely important that you are prepared for your interview. The interview process is an opportunity for the pharmacy technician and the employer to get to know each other, to determine whether you are the right employee for the position, and for you to discern whether the pharmacy meets your requirements.

It is extremely important for the pharmacy technician to be prepared for the interview. Being prepared includes wearing appropriate clothing for the interview, carrying oneself properly, answering questions asked by the interviewer, and asking questions of the interviewer. You will be assessed on what you do, what you say, and what you don't say. You will have only a few moments to impress the employer, so it is important to be prepared. Remember the saying, "Failing to prepare is preparing to fail."

Lab Activity #3.1: Mock interview

Equipment needed:

- Paper
- Pencil/pen

Time needed to complete this activity: 60 minutes

It is extremely important that you are prepared to answer any question that might be asked of you by the interviewer. Your response should be short and concise but should answer the question.

You are a pharmacy technician who has applied for a pharmacy technician position at a local pharmacy. The pharmacy has called and would like you to come in for an interview.

How would you answer the following questions?

1. Tell me about yourself.

_____

_____

2. Why did you decide to become a pharmacy technician?

_____

_____

3. Tell me about the pharmacy technician program that prepared you to become a pharmacy technician. What did you like about it? What did you dislike about it?

_____

_____

_____

_____

4. Did you have an externship? Where did you do your externship? How many hours was it?

_____

_____

5. Are you certified? If not, when will you be taking the test? Which test will you be taking?

_____

_____

6. Why will you be successful as a pharmacy technician?

_____

_____

7. Why do you want to work for us?

_____

_____

8. What do you know about our company?

_____

_____

9. Why should we hire you?

_____

_____

_____

10. What in your background prepares you for this job?

_____

_____

11. How will your job contribute to the overall goals of this company?

_____

_____

12. What do you think you're going to be doing for us?

_____

_____

13. What do you hope to be doing in 5 years?

_____

_____

14. How do you feel about what you've accomplished so far?

_____

_____

15. How do you work under pressure? Can you give us some examples?

_____

_____

_____

16. What is your greatest strength?

_____

_____

17. What is your greatest weakness? How have you overcome your weaknesses?

_____

_____

_____

_____

18. What do your references say about you?

_____

_____

19. Who was your best boss or manager? Why?

_____

_____

20. In your last job, what tasks took most of your time?

_____

_____

21. What did you enjoy doing most in your last job? Least?

_____

_____

_____

_____

22. How could you have improved your last job?

_____

_____

_____

23. Why did you leave your last job?

_____

_____

24. Have you ever had your work or your suggestions criticized or attacked? How did you react?

_____

_____

_____

25. What have you done that shows initiative?

_____

_____

26. Tell us about a time when you were completely committed.

_____

_____

27. Explain your role in a team. Tell us about something that you've accomplished working with others.

_____

_____

_____

28. Explain an event that challenged and changed you. Do you think your reaction to the event was different from other individuals?

_____

_____

29. What types of decisions or jobs give you trouble?

_____

_____

30. What skills do you need to improve upon the most? What are you doing to remedy that situation?

_____

_____

_____

31. What coursework have you completed that applies to this job?

_____

_____

32. How do you prefer to work: by yourself or with other people?

_____

_____

Chapter **3** **Pharmacy Ethics, Competencies**

During this part of the activity, act as if you are conducting an interview. Create interview questions for a classmate and rate their response. Also evaluate your classmate on attire, body language, and ability to answer questions. You may ask questions from the list above, or other questions that might be relevant during an interview.

Questions to Ask Interviewee	On a scale of 1 to 5, with "1" being the lowest and "5" being the highest, rate the potential employee's response to the question:
1.	
2.	
3.	
4.	
5.	
6.	
7.	
8.	
9.	
10.	
11.	
12.	
13.	
14.	
15.	

1. Would you hire the individual? Why or why not?

_____

_____

_____

Interview Evaluation	Yes/No
Prospective employee arrived on time for interview	
Employee introduced himself/herself to receptionist	
Completed an application legibly and did not leave questions unanswered	
Shook hands with the interviewer(s)	
Provided interviewer with a current resume	
Resumé was free of spelling and grammatical errors	
Prospective employee had a neat, clean appearance	
Interviewee wore appropriate clothes for an interview	

Interview Evaluation	Yes/No
Jewelry was appropriate for an interview	
Fragrance was subtle, not overwhelming	
Answered interview questions (behavioral and technical) appropriately	
Asked questions of the interviewer	
Thanked interviewer and shook hands as he/she was leaving	
Sent "Thank You" note to interviewer within 24 hours	

Pharmacy Technician Certification

Objective: To introduce the pharmacy technician to the process of becoming certified as a pharmacy technician in his/her state.

Certification is the process by which a government agency grants recognition to an individual who has met pre-determined qualifications specified by an agency or association. At the present moment, two pharmacy technician certification organizations are available: the Pharmacy Technician Certification Board (PTCB) and the Institute for Certification for Pharmacy Technicians (ICPT). Not all states require that a pharmacy technician is certified; however, there is a growing trend within the United States for pharmacy technicians to be certified as a prerequisite to working in a pharmacy, regardless of the setting.

Lab Activity #3.2: Visit *www.nabp.net* to obtain the website for your state board of pharmacy. After logging in to your state board of pharmacy, find out the requirements for a pharmacy technician to practice in your state. Complete the following table.

Equipment needed:

- Computer with Internet access
- Pencil/pen
- Paper

Time needed to complete this activity: 20 minutes

Question	Response
Name of state	
Does your state require pharmacy technicians to be certified?	
If yes, what certification tests are approved for your state?	
What is the fee for each test approved by your state?	
Does your state require licensure of pharmacy technicians?	
Is a fee required for licensure? If so, what is the fee? How often does a pharmacy technician need to renew his/her license?	
Does your state require pharmacy technicians to register with the state board of pharmacy?	

Question	Response
Is a fee associated with the registration? If yes, what is the fee?	
What continuing education does your state require of pharmacy technicians? Are continuing education requirements met on a yearly basis?	
What fees are required to be paid to the state board of pharmacy for technicians?	

Lab Activity #3.3: Visit *www.ptcb.org* and *www.nationaltechexam.org* to obtain information regarding each of these examinations. Complete the following table for each examination.

Equipment needed:

- Computer with Internet access

Time needed to complete this activity: 30 minutes

PTCB Examination	Response
What is the registration fee for the test?	
How often is the test offered?	
How many questions are included on the test?	
What is the minimum passing score for the examination?	
Where is the test offered in your area?	
If an individual does not pass the exam, when may he/she retake it?	
How long is the certification valid?	
How many continuing education units are required to renew your certification?	
Which states accept this exam?	

ExCPT Examination	Response
What is the registration fee for the test?	
How often is the test offered?	
How many questions are included on the test?	
What is the minimum passing score for the examination?	
If an individual does not pass the exam, when may he/she retake it?	
Where is the test offered in your area?	
How long is the certification valid?	
How many continuing education units are required to renew your certification?	
Which states accept this exam?	

Lab Activity #3.4: Print a copy of the content for the PTCB and ExCPT examinations. Compare and contrast the information included on each examination.

Equipment needed:

- Computer with Internet access
- Computer printer

Time to needed to complete this activity: 20 minutes

1. Which examination will you take and why?

_____

_____

_____

_____

_____

Lab Activity #3.5: Register for the PTCB exam or the ExCPT exam.

Equipment needed:

- Computer with Internet access
- Computer printer with paper
- Credit or debit card

Time needed to complete this activity: 20 minutes

1. When did you register?

_____

2. When are you scheduled to take the exam?

_____

3. Where are you to take the exam?

_____

Pharmacy Ethics

Objective: To identify those pharmacy situations in which a pharmacy technician will be faced with making ethical decisions.

The practice of pharmacy has established a code of ethics for both pharmacists and pharmacy technicians.

Code of Ethics for Pharmacy Technicians
Preamble
Pharmacy technicians are health care professionals who assist pharmacists in providing the best possible care for patients. The principles of this code, which apply to pharmacy technicians working in any and all settings, are based on application and support of the moral obligations that guide the pharmacy profession in relationships with patients, health care professionals, and society.

Principles
- A pharmacy technician's first consideration is to ensure the health and safety of the patient, and to use knowledge and skills to the best of his/her ability in serving patients.
- A pharmacy technician supports and promotes honesty and integrity in the profession, which includes the duty to observe the law, maintain the highest moral and ethical conduct at all times, and uphold the ethical principles of the profession.

- A pharmacy technician assists and supports pharmacists in the safe and efficacious and cost-effective distribution of health services and health care resources.
- A pharmacy technician respects and values the abilities of pharmacists, colleagues, and other health care professionals.
- A pharmacy technician maintains competency in his/her practice and continually enhances his/her professional knowledge and expertise.
- A pharmacy technician respects and supports the patient's individuality, dignity, and confidentiality.
- A pharmacy technician respects the confidentiality of a patient's records and discloses pertinent information only with proper authorization.
- A pharmacy technician never assists in dispensing, promoting, or distributing medication or medical devices that are not of good quality or that do not meet standards as required by law.
- A pharmacy technician does not engage in any activity that will discredit the profession, and will expose, without fear or favor, illegal or unethical conduct within the profession.
- A pharmacy technician associates with and engages in the support of organizations that promote the profession of pharmacy through the utilization and enhancement of pharmacy technicians.

Lab Activity #3.6: Explain how you would handle the following pharmacy situations and identify the principle of the code of ethics on which you are basing your decision.

Equipment needed:

- Pen/pencil

Time needed to complete the activity: 20 minutes

1. A friend of your family is diagnosed with a terminal illness and drops off a prescription to be filled. Should you tell your family about this individual's situation? Why or why not?

_____

_____

_____

2. You are not required to be certified as a pharmacy technician to practice in your state. Should you participate in continuing education activities? Why or why not?

_____

_____

_____

3. An individual wishes to purchase insulin syringes, and the pharmacist is not present in the pharmacy at that time. Should you sell the syringes to the customer or wait for the pharmacist to return? Why or why not?

_____

_____

_____

4. You have medication in your inventory that will expire in 8 days. A patient presents a prescription for a 10 days' supply of the medication. Should you dispense the medication on your shelf? Why or why not?

_____

_____

_____

5. You have dropped some medication on the floor. What should you do with this medication and why?

_____

_____

_____

6. A woman comes to the pharmacy and asks for a listing of the medications her husband filled last year. What should you do and why?

_____

_____

_____

7. A patient asks you to recommend an OTC medication for respiratory allergies. In the past, you have observed the pharmacist recommend Claritin; should you recommend Claritin to the patient? Why or why not?

_____

_____

_____

8. The FDA has recalled Drug X because of labeling problems, and you have some of the recalled medication on your shelf. An individual requests a refill for this medication on Friday and needs to leave on a plane in the afternoon. Should you dispense the recalled medication that is now on your shelf? Why or why not?

_____

_____

_____

9. You observe the pharmacist preparing an intravenous fluid at a strength that is less than what has been prescribed by the physician. How would you handle this situation?

_____

_____

_____

10. A physician had his license to prescribe medications suspended 5 years ago by both the board of medicine and the pharmacy because of a personal drug problem. His license to practice has been reinstated. A patient brings in a prescription from that physician and casually asks what you know about the physician. How would you handle the situation?

_____

_____

_____

Professionalism as a Pharmacy Technician

Objective: To become familiar with the professional organizations available for membership for pharmacy technicians and the resources that can be used to remain competent as a pharmacy technician.

Two of the principles of the Pharmacy Technician's Code of Ethics state the following:

- A pharmacy technician maintains competency in his/her practice, and continually enhances his/her professional knowledge and expertise.
- A pharmacy technician associates with and engages in the support of organizations that promote the profession of pharmacy through the utilization and enhancement of pharmacy technicians.

All certified pharmacy technicians are required to maintain their competency through continuing education. Continuing education may take the form of pharmacy seminars or workshops, webinars, or reading of print materials accredited by the ACPE.

A pharmacy technician should become involved with a pharmacy organization that will allow the pharmacy technician to develop professionally as a member of the organization. A pharmacy technician may choose to join many different types of organizations, depending on his/her interests. These organizations include the following:

- American Association of Pharmacy Technicians *(www.pharmacytechnician.com)*
- American Pharmacists Association *(www.pharmacist.com)*
- American Society of Health-System Pharmacists *(www.ashp.org)*
- National Pharmacy Technician Association *(www.pharmacytechnician.org)*
- Academy of Managed Care Pharmacy *(www.amcp.org)*

Lab Activity #3.7: Identify local, state, and national organizations that are available for membership for pharmacy technicians.

Equipment needed:

- Computer with Internet access
- Computer printer
- Paper
- Pencil/pen

Time needed to complete this activity: 20 minutes

Using the Internet, identify state and regional (local) pharmacy associations that you are eligible to join. Complete the following table.

Organization	Open to Pharmacy Technicians	Membership Fee	Continuing Education	Three Benefits of Membership	Career Opportunities
State association					
Regional association					
Academy of Managed Pharmacy *(www.amcp.org)*					
American Association of Pharmacy Technicians*(www.pharmacytechnician.com)*					

Organization	Open to Pharmacy Technicians	Membership Fee	Continuing Education	Three Benefits of Membership	Career Opportunities
American Pharmacist Association (www. pharmacist.com)					
American Society of Health-System Pharmacists (www. ashp.org)					
National Pharmacy Technician Association (www. pharmacytechnician.org)					

Lab Activity #3.8: Participate in pharmacy technician continuing education.

Equipment needed:
- Computer with Internet access
- Computer printer
- Paper
- Pencil/pen

Time needed to complete this activity: 1½ hours

Using the Internet, select a pharmacy continuing education article of your choice from one of the following websites.

- *www.freece.com*
- *www.modernmedicine.com*
- *www.pharmacychoice.com*
- *www.pharmacytimes.com*
- *www.powerpak.com*
- *www.rxschool.com*
- *www.rxschool.com*
- *www.uspharmacist.com*

Read the article, take the examination, and print out the continuing education certificate. Provide the certificate to your instructor.

4 Conversions and Calculations Used by Pharmacy Technicians

REINFORCE KEY CONCEPTS

TERMS AND DEFINITIONS

Select the correct term from the following list and write the corresponding letter in the blank next to the statement.

A. Allegation
B. Apothecary system
C. Avoirdupois system
D. International time
E. Metric system
F. Volume
G. Household
H. Diluent
I. Body surface area (BSA)
J. BSA nomogram

___C___ 1. A system of measurement based on multiples of 10

___H___ 2. An inert product, either liquid or solid, that is added to a preparation

___A___ 3. A method of determining the needed amounts of two different concentrations to prepare a needed concentration

___D___ 4. A 24-hour method of keeping time without distinguishing between AM and PM

___F___ 5. The amount of liquid enclosed in a container

___E___ 6. An English system of measurement used to determine weight

___J___ 7. Table used to determine a patient's body surface area

___B___ 8. A system of measurement used traditionally in pharmacy

___I___ 9. Used to provide an accurate dose for some medications based on both weight and height of the patient

___E___ 10. System of measurement customarily used in the United States for weight, volume, and length

TRUE OR FALSE

Write T or F next to each statement.

___T___ 1. The ability to manipulate conversions is a required competency of pharmacy technicians.

___F___ 2. Not all transcriptions and calculations need to be checked by a pharmacist.

___F___ 3. The *Apoth* metric system is used throughout pharmacy because it is the easiest to remember.

___T___ 4. All measurements used in pharmacy must be converted to the household system for the patient.

___T___ 5. Most pharmacy calculations are ratio-proportion equations.

___F___ 6. The *pharm* technician should show the parent of a pediatric patient how to measure the correct dosage.

___T___ 7. Many, but not all, IV piggyback solutions are given over 30 to 60 minutes.

___F___ 8. One of the most common errors made in pharmacy is placing a zero in front of a decimal.

___T___ 9. When conversion is done using the household system, the decimal must be moved to the right or to the left.

___F___ 10. Both Roman numerals and Arabic numbers are used in pharmacies.

___T___ 11. International time is also known as military time.

___F___ 12. It is not important for the technician to double-check the calculations because the pharmacist will check them.

MULTIPLE CHOICE

Complete each question by circling the best answer.

1. The cost of 100 g of hydrocortisone powder is $36.00. What would be the cost of 12 g?
   A. $5.42
   B. $4.32 $\frac{100}{36} \times \frac{12g}{x}$
   C. $10.60
   D. $8.94

2. A 125-pound patient weighs how many kilograms?
   A. 0.125
   B. 125,000 $2.2 \text{ lb} = 1 \text{ kg}$
   C. 56.82
   D. 275

3. Convert 1200 mg to grams.
   A. 12,000
   B. 12
   C. 120
   D. 1.2

4. Of the following, volume best refers to the measurement of:
   A. Liquids
   B. Dry ingredients
   C. Distance
   D. None of the above

5. The weight of 1 grain is:
   A. 60 mg
   B. 64 mg
   C. 65 mg
   D. All of the above; different measurement systems define grains in different weights

6. There are 1000 milligrams in 1
   A. Kilogram
   B. Gram
   C. Milligram
   D. Microgram

7. A freight box that weighs 633 kg weighs how many pounds?
   A. 0.633
   B. 1392.6
   C. 287.73
   D. 28.77

8. 25 teaspoons = _____ ml.

    A. 100

    B. 250

    C. 375

    Ⓓ. 125

9. A pharmacy wants to increase the price of a product by 35%. How much would an item cost with this markup if its original cost was $6.75?

    A. $6.95

    B. $8.21

    C. $12.50

    Ⓓ. $9.11

10. The approximate size of a container used to dispense 120 ml of a liquid medication would be:

    Ⓐ. 6 oz

    B. 4 oz

    C. 8 oz

    D. 2 oz

11. A physician orders ampicillin 0.5 g PO q6h. The medication available is ampicillin 125 mg/5 ml. What is the quantity of medication to be administered per dose? administered ? = 1 dose

    Ⓐ. 20 ml $\frac{0.500 mg}{x\,ml} \times \frac{125\,mg}{1\,mL}$

    B. 2 ml

    C. 0.2 ml

    D. 0.02 ml

12. The physician orders atropine 1/150 gr PO bid. The atropine available is 0.4 mg per tablet. The nurse will administer how many tablets per dose? (use 60 mg/gr)

    A. 0.5

    Ⓑ. 0.75

    C. 1

    D. 1.5

13. A prescription is written for Pen VK 500 mg tabs PO qid for 10 days. The patient, who has throat cancer and cannot swallow, requests a liquid form. What volume of a 250 mg/5 ml suspension should be dispensed to fill the prescription?

    Ⓐ. 40 ml

    B. 400 ml

    C. 150 ml

    D. 250 ml

14. A pharmacist dispenses 300 ml of amoxicillin 150 mg/5 ml suspension. The sig is 250 mg PO tid mcg. How many days will the prescription last?

    A. 7

    B. 10

    Ⓒ. 12

    D. 14

Chapter **4** **Conversions and Calculations Used by Pharmacy Technicians**

15. The physician's order is for Timoptic ii gtts ou bid. How many drops will the patient get in 12 days?
    A. 4
    B. 48
    C. 69
    D. 96

16. You receive an order for Kaopectate 15 ml bid prn. One dose equals how many tablespoonfuls?
    A. 2
    B. 3
    C. 1
    D. 1.5

17. Mylanta and Donnatal are to be combined in a 2:1 ratio. How many milliliters of each is required to make 120 ml of the suspension?
    A. 70 ml/50 ml
    B. 50 ml/70 ml
    C. 80 ml/40 ml
    D. 40 ml/80 ml

18. An IV solution is ordered to run at 3.5 gtts/min. It contains 875 mg in a total of 250 ml. How many milligrams will the patient receive per hour if the set is calibrated to deliver 12 gtts/ml?
    A. 0.16 mg/hr
    B. 16 mg/hr
    C. 61.25 mg/hr
    D. 610 mg/hr

19. The Roman numeral XLVIII is equivalent to:
    A. 43
    B. 48
    C. 53
    D. 58

20. Convert 12:14 AM to military (international) time.
    A. 1214
    B. 0214
    C. 0014
    D. 0140

21. The Roman numeral LVIII is equivalent to:
    A. 58
    B. 48
    C. 38
    D. 68

22. How many days will the following prescription last? Zoloft 100 mg #90
    Sig: 1 PO bid
    A. 55
    B. 30
    C. 45
    D. 90

40

23. A dose is written for 10 mg/kg every 12 hours for 1 day. The adult taking this medication weighs 165 pounds. How much drug will be needed for this order?

    A. 425 mg

    B. 950 mg

    C. 750 mg

    D. 1500 mg

24. How many tablets would be needed for the following prescription?

    Prednisone tablets 10 mg

    One qid for 6 days; one tid for 3 days; one bid for 1 day; then stop

    A. 35

    B. 15

    C. 25

    D. 45

25. Using the following DEA formula, what should be the last digit of this DEA number?

    AB461853 _____

    DEA formula: Add 1st+3rd+5th numbers = _____

    Add 2nd+4th+6th numbers = then multiply by 2 = _____

    Add the two sums together; the last digit on the right should be the last digit of the number:

    A. 7

    B. 4

    C. 2

    D. 8

26. A dosage of 0.5 g is prescribed. You have in stock 150 mg/ml. How many milliliters would be given using the dosage strength on hand?

    A. 2

    B. 5

    C. 3.3

    D. 1.5

27. How many milligrams of epinephrine is needed to prepare 3 L of a 1:30,000 solution?

    A. 0.1

    B. 1

    C. 10

    D. 100

28. How many liters of a 0.9% normal saline solution can be made from 60 g of NaCl?

    A. 6.67

    B. 66.7

    C. 667

    D. 6667

Chapter **4** **Conversions and Calculations Used by Pharmacy Technicians**

29. If 5 ml of diluent is added to a vial containing 2 g of a drug for injection, resulting in a final volume of 5.8 ml, what is the concentration in milligrams per milliliters of the drug in the reconstituted solution? PV

    A. 0.3 mg/ml

    B. 345 mg/ml

    C. 444 mg/ml

    D. 2035 mg/ml

30. Which prescription instructions would require 21 tablets to be dispensed?

    A. One tab PO bid for 8 d

    B. One tab ac hs for 4 d

    C. One tab tid for 3 d; one tab bid for 3 d; one qd for 3 d

    D. Three tabs bid for 2 d; two tabs qd for 3 d; one tab qd for 3 d

31. How many grams of potassium permanganate is required to prepare 2 quarts of a 1:750 solution of potassium permanganate?

    A. 1.28

    B. 3

    C. 2.56

    D. 5

32. If the dosage of a drug is 35 mg/kg/day in six divided doses, how much would be given in each dose to a 38-pound child?

    A. 17.3 mg

    B. 60.4 mg

    C. 101 mg

    D. 604 mg

33. To make 300 ml of a 5% dextrose solution, using 10% dextrose solution and water, how much of each do you need? (Use the allegation method.)

    A. 150 ml dextrose 10% solution and 150 ml water

    B. 175 ml dextrose 10% solution and 125 ml water

    C. 180 ml dextrose 10% solution and 120 ml water

    D. 200 ml dextrose 10% solution and 100 ml water

34. How many capsules, each containing 1.5 gr of a drug, can be filled completely from a 28 g bottle of the drug? (Use 60 mg/gr.)

    A. 24

    B. 32

    C. 311

    D. 431

35. An IV solution containing 20,000 units of heparin in 500 ml of 0.45% NaCl solution is to be infused to provide 1000 units of heparin per hour. Roughly how many drops per minute should be infused to deliver the desired dose if the IV set calibrates at 15 gtt/ml?

    A. 0.42 gtt/min

    B. 6 gtt/min

    C. 16 gtt/min

    D. 32 gtt/min

CONVERSIONS

Convert the following measurements:

1. 8 ounces = _240_ ml
2. 90 ml = _3_ oz
3. 3 kg = _3000_ g
4. 2 pints = _4_ cups
5. 3.5 = _0.035_ % 350
6. 0.25 = _25_ %
7. 1.5 gr = _1500_ mg 10
8. 55 lb = _121_ kg 25
9. 125 kg = _57_ lb 257
10. 2500 ml = _2.5_ L
11. 0.15 mg = _150_ mcg
12. 3600 ml = _6_ pts 7.5
13. 78 mg = _1.3_ gr
14. 33% = _0.33_ decimal
15. 40% = _.40_ decimal

Convert the following Roman numerals to Arabic and Arabic to Roman:

1. XV _____
2. XCIV _____
3. 250 _____
4. 49 _____
5. MDX _____
6. XXXIII _____
7. 125 _____
8. 60 _____
9. IX _____
10. CC _____

SHORT ANSWER

Write a short response to each question in the space provided.

1. Give the units used in the metric system for the following:
   A. Volume

   _____

   B. Weight

   _____

   C. Distance

   _____

2. Give the units used in the household system for the following:
   A. Volume

   _____

   B. Weight

   _____

   C. Distance

   _____

Chapter **4** **Conversions and Calculations Used by Pharmacy Technicians**

3. Give the units used in the apothecary system for the following:

   A. Liquids

   _____

   B. Dry weights

   _____

4. Give the units used in the Avoirdupois system for the following:

   A. Liquids

   _____

   B. Weights

   _____

REFLECT CRITICALLY

CRITICAL THINKING

Reply to each question based on what you have learned in the chapter.

1. Bobbi is a second semester pharmacy technician student. She is having difficulty with her calculations course. Although the instructor assures her it is necessary to have a solid working knowledge of pharmacy math, she is not sure she will really ever have to use it on the job. How would you convince Bobbi of the importance of a strong calculations foundation?

   Show her some calculations that she would have to do on the job. It is essential to be able to do conversions and calculations. In some cases it is life or death.

2. Proper decimal notation is crucial in pharmacy calculations, and technicians cannot afford to misread a prescription. What would be the outcome if a pharmacy technician mistook 5 mcg for 5 mg and the pharmacist did not catch the error?

   The patient would die perhaps or be on another drug - not overdose wt maybe not have symptoms alleviated.

3. A compounding pharmacy receives an order for a 1% ointment. The technician weighs out 2 g of the active ingredient. What is the final weight of the correctly compounded prescription?

   $\frac{1g}{100g} \times \frac{2g}{xg}$ *200g for 1%.* $\frac{2g}{200g}$ *is 1% strength*

4. A technician is filling a medication for a 4-year-old child. The average adult dose is 250 mg. How much medication should the child receive?

   $\frac{250 mg}{4} = 62.5$. *Divide the dosage into 1/4 original and give accordingly.*

LAB SCENARIOS

Pharmacy Conversions

Objective: To introduce and review various pharmacy math conversions with the pharmacy technician.

Prescribers write prescriptions and medication orders using a variety of measurement systems, which include metric, household, apothecary, and avoirdupois systems. The metric system is the legal standard of measure in the United States, and other systems are referred to it for official comparison. Two advantages of the metric system are (1) that its tables are simple to understand because they are based on the decimal system, and (2) that the greater of two consecutive denominations is always 10 times the lesser amount.

The basic units of measurements of the metric system are as follows:

- The meter for length
- The liter for volume
- The gram for weight

The United States Pharmacopeia (USP) has established the metric system as the approved system of measurement in the United States. However, the pharmacy technician must be familiar with the other systems of measurements when interpreting prescription and medication orders.

Lab Activity #4.1: Identify the meaning of the following metric prefixes.

Equipment needed:

- Pen/pencil

Time needed to complete this activity: 5 minutes

1. micro- _____

2. milli- _____

3. centi- _____

4. deci- _____

5. deka- _____

6. hecto- _____

7. kilo- _____

Lab Activity #4.2: Convert the following measurement system to the measurement system used in the practice of pharmacy.

Equipment needed:

- Pen/pencil
- Calculator

Time needed to complete this activity: 30 minutes

1. 250 mcg   =   _____ mg

2. 100 mg   =   _____ g

3. 10 g   =   _____ mg

4. 12 fl oz   =   _____ pt

5. 2 pt   =   _____ gal

6. 2500 g   =   _____ kg

7. 10 tbsp   =   _____ fl oz

8. 480 ml   =   _____ qt

9. 5 kg   =   _____ g

10. 12 tsp   =   _____ tbsp

11. 3 gr   =   _____ mg

12. 144 tsp   =   _____ gal

13. 6 tbsp   =   _____ ml

14. 1500 mcg   =   _____ g

15. 30 ml   =   _____ tsp

16. 6 fl oz   =   _____ tsp

17. 12 fl oz   =   _____ cup

18. 0.4 kg   =   _____ mg

Chapter **4** **Conversions and Calculations Used by Pharmacy Technicians**

5 mL = 1 tsp
3 tsp = 1 tbsp
2 tbsp fl oz
2 =1 cup
3 oz = 1 cup
cups pint
2 pints quart
2 pints = 1 qt
4 quarts = 1 gal

19. 360 ml   =   1.5   cup

20. 0.5 g   =   500,600   mcg

21. 480 ml   =   0.125 gal   0·125

22. 8 tsp   =   40   ml

23. 0.1 mg   =   100   mcg   6 tsp1 oz   8 oz/1 cup

24. 1 pt   =   96   tsp   2 cups = 1 pt

25. 12 tsp   =   0.25 cup   16 oz   4 tbsp → 2 oz

26. 720 ml   =   1.5 pt   16 oz = 1 pt   480 ml

27. 32 fl oz   =   _____ qt

28. 325 mg   =   _____ gr

29. 48 tsp   =   _____ pt

30. 1 cup   =   _____ pt

31. 12 tbsp   =   _____ tsp

32. 120 ml   =   _____ fl oz

33. 4 cup   =   _____ gal

34. 24 tsp   =   _____ fl oz

35. 4 pt   =   _____ qt

36. 24 tbsp   =   _____ cup

37. 4 fl oz   =   _____ ml

38. 90 ml   =   _____ tbsp

39. 8 fl oz   =   _____ tbsp

40. 0.5 kg   =   _____ mcg

41. 64 fl oz   =   _____ gal

42. 2 cup   =   _____ ml

43. 0.5 gal   =   _____ pt

44. 0.5 cup   =   _____ tbsp

45. 1 qt   =   _____ fl oz

46. 1 cup   =   _____ fl oz

47. 96 tbsp   =   _____ qt

48. 0.25 gal   =   _____ fl oz

49. 2 cup   =   _____ qt

50. 96 tsp   =   _____ qt

51. 2 pt   =   _____ ml

52. 1 pt   =   _____ fl oz

53. 1 cup   =   _____ tsp

54. 2 pt   =   _____ cup

55. 2 gal   =   _____ cup

56. 2 qt   =   _____ ml

57. 1.5 qt   =   _____ tsp

58. 1 qt   =   _____ tbsp

59. 2 qt   =   _____ pt

60. 1 qt   =   _____ gal

61. 2 gal   =   _____ ml

62. 0.25 gal   =   _____ tsp

63. 1 gal   =   _____ tbsp

64. 8 pt   =   _____ tbsp

65. 48 tbsp   =   _____ pt

66. 1 gal   =   _____ qt

Reducing and Enlarging a Formula

Objective: To introduce and review with the pharmacy technician the steps needed to enlarge or reduce a prescription.

A pharmacy technician may receive a prescription or medication that requires enlargement or reduction of the formula for a compound. The technician may be required to calculate the quantity of each ingredient in the compound. A formula may be expressed in specific quantities for each ingredient or in parts. To enlarge or reduce a formula using specific quantities, the following formula may be used:

$$\frac{\text{Total quantity of formula (as specified)}}{\text{Total quantity of formula (as desired)}} = \frac{\text{Quantity of an ingredient (as specified in formula)}}{X}$$

where X = quantity of an ingredient for the quantity desired
   If the order is written using parts, the following formula can be used:

$$\frac{\text{Total number of parts in formula (as specified)}}{\text{Number of parts of an ingredient (as specified)}} = \frac{\text{Total quantity of formula (as desired)}}{X \text{ (quantity of an ingredient)}}$$

Chapter **4**   **Conversions and Calculations Used by Pharmacy Technicians**

Lab Activity #4.3: Reducing and enlarging a prescription. Calculate the correct quantities of each ingredient needed to prepare the following compounds.

Equipment needed:

- Pen/pencil
- Calculator

Time needed to complete this activity: 30 min

1. Following is the formula to compound 1000 g of Yellow Ointment, USP:

   Yellow Wax   50 g

   Petrolatum   950 g

   How much of each ingredient should be used to prepare 2 ounces of Yellow Ointment, USP?

   Yellow Wax   _____

   Petrolatum   _____

2. Following is the formula for Calamine Lotion:

   Calamine   80 g → $\frac{80\ gm}{1000\ ml} \times \frac{x\ g}{240\ ml} = 19.2\ g$

   Zinc Oxide   80 g → $\frac{80\ gm}{1000\ ml} \times \frac{x\ g}{240\ ml} = SAME$ Glycerin $\frac{20g}{1000ml} \times \frac{x}{240}$

   Glycerin   20 g

   Bentonite Magma   250 ml → $\frac{250\ ml}{1000ml}$ & $\frac{x\ ml}{480ml}$

   Calcium Hydroxide qs to   1000 ml   — (perfect Liter)

   How much of each ingredient should be used to prepare 8 fluid ounces of Calamine Lotion?

   Calamine   8%   { 19.2 g   (240 ml)   Lot #'s / Exp Dates

   Zinc Oxide   8%   { 19.2 g } 43.2 g

   Glycerin   2%   { 4.8 g

   Bentonite Magma   25%   45.2 ml 60 ml → 103.2 = TV

   Calcium Hydroxide   qs to   136.8 ml → (240 ml)
             volume desired

3. Following is the formula for Benzoin Tincture Compound:

   Benzoin   100 g $\frac{100g}{1000ml} \times \frac{x}{960ml}$ =

   Aloe   20 g $\frac{20g}{1000ml} \times \frac{x}{960\ ml}$

   Storax   80 g → $\frac{80\ g}{1000\ ml} \times \frac{x}{960}$ =

   Tolu Balsam   40 g

   Alcohol qs   1000 ml   960 mL

   How much of each ingredient should be used in this preparation to make one quart of Benzoin Tincture Compound?

   Benzoin   10%   _____96 g_____

   Aloe   2%   _____19.2 g_____

   Storax   8%   _____76.8 g_____

   Tolu Balsam   4%   _____38.4 g_____

   Alcohol qs   _____729.6 mL qs_____

    Chapter **4** **Conversions and Calculations Used by Pharmacy Technicians**

[Handwritten notes at top left margin]
CT - 6%.
20 - 2%.
Ho -
pylene
glycol
month
piration
date

[Handwritten calculations at top]
2 oz 6 × ×gm 3.6 gm 4.8 mL
     100   60g
     2/100 × ×gm = 1.2 gm 2mL glycol
            600m
     TV = 7.8 mL - 60gm = 52.2g
                    Ho
CT → 5/65 × ×gm/454g = 34.92 gm
ZO = 10/65 × gm/454 = 69.85 gm
Ho :

4. Following is the formula for Coal Tar Ointment:

Coal Tar   5 parts   *65 total parts*

Zinc Oxide   10 parts   *manufacturing pound*

Hydrophilic Ointment   50 parts *solvent, vehicle*   *vs pharmacy pound = 480 lbs compounding*

How much of each ingredient should be used to make one pound of Coal Tar Ointment?   *454 gm*

Coal Tar   *34.92 gm*

Zinc Oxide   *69.85 gm*

Hydrophilic Ointment   *349.23 gm*

5. Following is the formula to prepare 1000 g of Hydrophilic Petrolatum, USP:

Cholesterol   30 g

Stearyl Alcohol   30 g

White Wax   80 g

White Petrolatum   860 g

How much of each ingredient should be used to prepare ½ pound of Hydrophilic Petrolatum, USP?

Cholesterol   _____

Stearyl Alcohol   _____

White Wax   _____

White Petrolatum   _____

6. Following is the formula to prepare 1000 g of Hydrophilic Ointment, USP:

Methylparaben   0.25 g

Propylparaben   0.15 g

Sodium Lauryl Sulfate   10 g

Propylene Glycol   120 g

Stearyl Alcohol   250 g

White Petrolatum   250 g

Purified Water   370 g

How much of each ingredient should be used to prepare 4 oz of Hydrophilic Ointment, USP?

Methylparaben   _____

Propylparaben   _____

Sodium Lauryl Sulfate   _____

Propylene Glycol   _____

Stearyl Alcohol   _____

White Petrolatum   _____

Purified Water   _____

7. Following is the formula to prepare 1000 ml of Benzyl Benzoate Lotion:

Benzyl Benzoate   250 ml

Triethanolamine   5 ml

Oleic Acid   20 ml

Purified Water qs   1000 ml

How much of each ingredient should be used to prepare one pint of Benzyl Benzoate Lotion?

Benzyl Benzoate   _____

Triethanolamine   _____

Oleic Acid   _____

Purified Water qs   _____

8. Following is the formula to prepare 1000 ml of Phenobarbital Elixir:

Phenobarbital	4 g
Orange Oil	0.25 ml
Certified Red Color	qs
Alcohol	200 ml
Propylene Glycol	100 ml
Sorbitol Solution	600 ml
Water qs	1000 ml

How much of each ingredient should be used to prepare 2 gallons of Phenobarbital Elixir?

Phenobarbital   _____

Orange Oil   _____

Certified Red Color   _____

Alcohol   _____

Propylene Glycol   _____

Sorbitol Solution   _____

Water qs   _____

9. Following is the formula to prepare 1 liter of White Lotion, USP:

Zinc Sulfate	40 g
Sulfurated Potash	40 g
Purified Water ad	1000 ml

How much of each ingredient should be used to prepare 1 cup of White Lotion, USP?

Zinc Sulfate   _____

Sulfurated Potash   _____

Purified Water ad   _____

10. Following is the formula to prepare 1 liter of Iodine Topical Solution, USP:

Iodine	20 g
Sodium Iodide	24 g
Purified Water ad	1000 ml

How much of each ingredient should be used to prepare sixty 15-ml bottles of Iodine Topical Solution, USP?

Iodine   _____

Sodium Iodide   _____

Purified Water ad   _____

Chapter **4** **Conversions and Calculations Used by Pharmacy Technicians**

Medication Concentrations (Strengths)

Objective: To become familiar with the concepts of percent weight-weight, weight-volume, and volume-volume.

A medication's concentration (strength) can be expressed mathematically in several different manners, which include a fraction, a ratio, or a percent. The term *percent* or its corresponding sign (%) means "by the hundred," and percentage means "rate per 100." A percent may also be expressed as a ratio represented as a common or decimal fraction. Percents are usually changed to equivalent decimal fractions. This change is made by dropping the percent sign (%) and dividing the expressed numerator by a fraction.

A medication expressed as a percent can be a solid dissolved in another solid, a solid dissolved in a liquid, or a liquid dissolved in another liquid.

- w/w% is defined as the number of grams of solute dissolved in 100 grams of vehicle base.
- w/v% is defined as the number of grams of solute dissolved in 100 milliliters of vehicle base.
- v/v% is defined as the number of milliliters of solute dissolved in 100 milliliters of vehicle base.

The following formula can be used in calculating the amount of solute, the total amount of vehicle base, or its percent.

$$\frac{\text{Amount of solute}}{\text{Amount of vehicle base}} = \frac{\%}{100}$$

The concentration of a weak solution or liquid preparation is frequently expressed in terms of ratio strength. Because all percentages represent a ratio of parts per hundred, ratio strength is another way of expressing the percentage strength of solutions or liquid preparations. For example, 10% means 10 parts per 100 or 10:100. Although 10 parts per 100 designates a ratio strength, it is customary to translate the designation into a ratio of one; therefore, 10:100 = 1:10.

When a ratio strength is used to designate a concentration, it is to be interpreted as the following:

- For solids in liquids = 1 g of solute in 1000 ml of solution or liquid preparation
- For liquids in liquids = 1 ml of solute in 1000 ml of solution or liquid preparation
- For solids in solids = 1 g of solute in 1000 g of mixture

The following formula can be used to calculate the number of parts, the total number of parts, or the percent of a ratio strength problem:

$$\frac{\text{\# parts}}{\text{Total parts}} \qquad \frac{\%}{100\%}$$

Lab Activity #4.4: In the following table, convert the following percent strength to ratio strength and ratio strength to percent strength.

Equipment needed:

- Calculator
- Pencil/pen

Time needed to complete this activity: 10 minutes

Percent Strength	Ratio Strength
25%	
	1:200
15%	
	1:400
50%	
	1:150

Percent Strength	Ratio Strength
4%	
	1:500
2%	
	1:175

Lab Activity #4.5: Solve the following problems involving percent strength and ratio strength.

Equipment needed:

- Calculator
- Pencil/pen
- Paper

Time needed to complete this activity: 45 minutes

Rx   Antipyrine   5%

Glycerin   ad   60 ml

Sig: gtt v in right ear tid

1. How many grams of antipyrine should be used in preparing the prescription?

   _____

   Rx   Resin of Podophyllum   25%

   Compound Benzoin Tincture   ad   30 ml

   Sig: Apply to papillomas tid

2. How many grams of resin of podophyllum should be used in preparing the prescription?

   _____

   Rx   Potassium Iodide Solution   10%

   Ephedrine Sulfate Solution   3%   aa 15 ml

   Sig: Place five drops in water as directed

3. How many grams of potassium iodide and ephedrine sulfate should be used in preparing the prescription?

   _____

   Rx   Iodochlorhydroxyquin   0.9 g

   Hydrocortisone   0.15 g

   Cream Base   ad   30 g

   Sig: Apply to the affected areas of skin once a day.

4. What is the percentage strength (w/w) each of iodochlohydroxyquin and hydrocortisone in the prescription?

   _____

5. How many milligrams of methylparaben are needed to prepare 16 fluid ounces of a solution containing 0.12% (w/v) of methylparaben?

   _____

6. A formula for a mouth rinse contains 1/10% (w/v) of zinc chloride. How many grams of zinc chloride should be used in preparing 20 liters of the mouth rinse?

   _____

     Chapter **4** **Conversions and Calculations Used by Pharmacy Technicians**

7. If 425 g of sucrose is dissolved in enough water to make 500 ml, what is the percentage strength (w/v) of the solution?

_____

8. How many milliliters of 0.9% (w/v) sodium chloride solution can be made from 1 lb of sodium chloride?

_____

9. One gallon of a certain lotion contains 946 ml of benzyl benzoate. Calculate the percentage (v/v) of benzyl benzoate in the lotion.

_____

10. A liniment contains 15% of methyl salicylate. How many milliliters of the liniment can be made from 1 quart of methyl salicylate?

_____

11. How many grams each of resorcinol and hexachlorophene should be used in preparing 2 pounds of an acne ointment that is to contain 2% resorcinol and 0.25% of hexachlorophene?

_____

12. How many milligrams of procaine hydrochloride should be used in preparing 60 suppositories, each weighing 2 grams and containing ¼% of procaine hydrochloride?

_____

13. If a topical cream contains 1.8% (w/w) of hydrocortisone, how many milligrams of hydrocortisone should be used in preparing 1 ounce of the cream?

_____

14. A pharmacist incorporates 6 grams of coal tar into 120 grams of a 6% coal tar ointment. Calculate the percentage (w/w) of coal tar in the finished product.

_____

15. Express each of the following concentrations as a ratio strength:

a. 2 mg of active ingredient in ml of solution _____

b. 0.275 mg of active ingredient in 5 ml of solution _____

c. 2 g of active ingredient in 250 ml of solution _____

d. 1 mg of active ingredient in 0.5 ml of solution _____

16. A vaginal cream contains 0.01% (w/v) of dienestrol. Express this concentration as a ratio strength.

_____

Rx	Menthol	1:500
	Hexachlorophene	1:800
	Hydrophilic Ointment Base	ad	60 g
	Sig: Apply to hands bid	

17. How many milligrams each of menthol and hexachlorophene should be used in compounding the prescription?

_____

18. Hepatitis B Virus Vaccine Inactivated is inactivated with 1:4000 (w/v) of formalin. Express this ratio strength as a percentage strength.

_____

19. Versed Injection contains 5 mg of midazolam per milliliter of injection. Calculate the ratio strength of midazolam in the injection.

_____

20. A sample of white petrolatum contains 10 mg of tocopherol per kilogram as a preservative. Express the amount of tocopherol as a ratio strength.

_____

Dilution Calculations

Objective: To become familiar with calculations used in the dilution of a product.

A pharmacy may receive a prescription for a medication in which the prescribed concentration is less than what is currently stocked in the pharmacy. The concentration may be written in the form of a percent, fraction, or ratio. In a dilution problem, the initial strength (the stock strength) is greater than the final strength (the prescribed strength). A diluent (an inert substance that does not have strength) is added to the initial volume or weight to make the final volume or weight. In other words, the amount of diluent can be calculated by using the following formula:

Final volume (weight) − Initial volume (weight) = Amount of diluent to be added

A dilution problem may be solved using the following formula:

(Initial strength) (Initial volume) = (Final strength) (Final volume)

or

(Initial strength) (Initial weight) = (Final strength) (Final weight)

It is important to remember that both initial and final strengths may be expressed in the same concentration, and that initial and final volumes (weight) may be expressed in the same unit of measurement.

Lab Activity #4.6: Calculate the quantity of the ingredient needed to prepare the following prescriptions.

Equipment needed:

- Calculator
- Pencil/pen
- Paper

Time to complete this activity: 30 minutes

1. Rx 1:

Dr. Andrew A. Sheen
1100 Brentwood Blvd, Suite M780
St. Louis, MO 63144
314-527-0000
DEA FS1234563

Dr. Andrew A. Sheen   January 12, 201X
1100 Brentwood Blvd Suite M780   St. Louis, MO 63144

FOR OFFICE USE

Rx   Isopropyl Alcohol 30%   1 gallon
      To be used in office for soaking sponges

Ref   Dr. Andrew Sheen

The pharmacy has in stock Isopropyl 70%. How much of the 70% concentration and diluent is needed to prepare this prescription?

Isopropyl Alcohol 30%: _____

Diluent: _____

Chapter **4** **Conversions and Calculations Used by Pharmacy Technicians**

2. Rx 2:

```
                        Dr. Andrew A. Sheen
                     1100 Brentwood Blvd, Suite M780
                          St. Louis, MO 63144
                             314-527-0000
                            DEA FS1234563


Dr. Andrew A. Sheen                              January 12, 201X
1100 Brentwood Blvd Suite M780                   St. Louis, MO 63144

                          FOR OFFICE USE

Rx      Zephiran 7.5%      1 gallon
        For office use

Ref                                  Dr. Andrew Sheen
```

The pharmacy has in stock Zephiran Chloride 20%. How much of the 20% Zephiran Chloride and diluent is needed to prepare this prescription?

Zephiran Chloride 20%: _____

Diluent: _____

3. Rx 3:

```
                        Dr. Andrew A. Sheen
                     1100 Brentwood Blvd, Suite M780
                          St. Louis, MO 63144
                             314-527-0000
                            DEA FS1234563

Dr. Andrew A. Sheen                              January 12, 201X
1100 Brentwood Blvd Suite M780                   St. Louis, MO 63144

                          FOR OFFICE USE

Rx      Hypochlorous acid 1:10    4 liters
        For office use

Ref                                  Dr. Andrew Sheen
```

The pharmacy has in stock 25% Hypochlorous Acid. How much of the 25% Hypochlorous Acid and diluent is needed to prepare this order?

Hypochlorous Acid 25%: _____

Diluent: _____

Rx   Gentian Violet Solution   1:100,000   500 ml

Sig: Use as a mouthwash

4. How many milliliters of a ½% solution of gentian violet should be used in preparing the prescription?
_____

Rx   Benzalkonium Chloride Solution   240 ml

Make a solution such that 10 ml diluted to a liter equals a 1:5000 solution

Sig: 10 ml diluted to a liter for external use

5. How many milliliters of a 17% solution of benzalkonium chloride should be used in preparing the prescription?
_____

6. How many milliliters of a 1:50 (w/v) boric acid solution can be prepared from 500 ml of a 5% (w/v) boric acid solution?
_____

7. How many milliliters of water must be added to 250 ml of a 25% (w/v) stock solution of sodium chloride to prepare a 0.9% (w/v) sodium chloride solution?

_____

8. How many milliliters of a 1% (w/v) solution of phenyl mercuric nitrate may be used in preparing a 100-ml prescription requiring 1:50,000 (w/v) of phenyl mercuric nitrate as a preservative?

_____

9. How many milliliters of water should be added to 1gallon of 70% isopropyl alcohol to prepare a 30% solution for soaking sponges?

_____

10. How many milliliters of water should be added to a liter of 1:3000 (w/v) solution to make a 1:8000 (w/v) solution?

_____

11. How many milliliters of water for injection must be added to 10 liters of a 50% (w/v) dextrose injection to reduce the concentration to 30% (w/v)?

_____

12. A physician orders 1 pint of 10% ethyl alcohol. The stock solution is 200 ml of 95% ethyl alcohol. How many milliliters of the 95% stock solution would be necessary to prepare the 10% solution?

_____

13. The pharmacy has 300 ml of a 50% solution. 200 ml is added to this solution to reduce the concentration. How many grams of active ingredient would be included in 4 fluid ounces of the diluted solution?

_____

14. How many grams of salicylic acid should be added to 75 g of a polyethylene glycol ointment to prepare an ointment containing 6% (w/w) of salicylic acid?

_____

15. How many grams of petrolatum (diluent) should be added to 250 g of a 255 ichthammol ointment to make a 5% ointment?

_____

Lab Activity #4.7: Calculate the final strength of the compound to appear on the prescription label from the following prescription.

Equipment needed:

- Calculator
- Pencil/pen
- Paper

Time needed to complete this activity: 30 minutes

1. If 250 ml of a 1/800 (v/v) solution is diluted to 1 liter, what will be the ratio strength (v/v)?

_____

2. Aluminum acetate topical solution contains 5% (w/v) of aluminum acetate. When 100 ml is diluted to a ½ liter, what will be the ratio strength?

_____

3. If 500 ml of a 10% (w/v) solution is diluted to 2 liters, what will be the percentage strength (w/v)?

_____

Chapter **4** **Conversions and Calculations Used by Pharmacy Technicians**

4. If 2 tablespoonfuls of povidone-iodine solution (10% w/v) is diluted to 1 quart with purified water, what is the ratio strength of the dilution?

_____

5. If 400 ml of a 20% (w/v) solution is diluted to 2 liters, what will be the percentage strength?

_____

6. If a 0.067% (w/v) methylbenzethonium chloride lotion is diluted with an equal volume of water, what will be the ratio strength (w/v) of the dilution?

_____

7. In preparing a solution for a wet dressing, two 0.3-g tablets of potassium permanganate are dissolved in 1 gallon of purified water. What will be the percentage strength (w/v) of the solution?

_____

8. If 150 ml of a 17% (w/v) concentrate of benzalkonium chloride is diluted to 5 gallons, what will be the ratio strength?

_____

9. If a pharmacy technician adds 3 g of hydrocortisone to 60 g of a 5% (w/w) hydrocortisone cream, what is the final percentage strength of hydrocortisone in the product?

_____

10. If 20 ml of a 2% (w/v) solution is diluted with water to 8 pints, what is the ratio strength (w/v) of the solution?

_____

Allegation Calculations

Objective: Perform pharmacy calculations using both allegation medial and allegation alternate in compounding prescriptions with multiple strengths of a medication.

Allegation medial is a method by which the "weighted average" percentage strength of a mixture of two or more substances of known quantity and concentration may be easily calculated. By this method, the percentage strength of each component expressed as a decimal fraction is multiplied by its corresponding quantity; then the sum of the products is divided by the total quantity of the mixture, and the resultant decimal fraction is multiplied by 100 to give the percentage of the mixture. Allegation medial can be used with both solids and liquids.

For example, consider the following problem. What is the percentage strength in a mixture of 300 ml of a 40% (v/v) alcohol, 100 ml of a 60% (v/v) alcohol, and 100 ml of a 70% alcohol?

$$0.4 \times 300\,ml = 120\,ml$$
$$0.6 \times 100\,ml = 60\,ml$$
$$\underline{0.7 \times 100\,ml = 70\,ml}$$
$$\text{Totals: } 500\,ml = 250\,ml$$
$$250\,ml/500\,ml = 0.5$$
$$0.5 \times 100 = 50\%$$

Allegation alternate is a method by which we calculate the number of parts of two or more components of a given strength when they are mixed to prepare a mixture of desired strength. The desired strength of the compound is between the strengths of the two medications on hand.

Lab Activity #4.8: Practice pharmacy calculations using allegation medial and allegation alternate.

Equipment needed:

- Calculator
- Pencil/pen
- Paper

Time needed to complete this activity: 30 minutes

1. Four equal amounts of belladonna extract, containing 1.15%, 1.3%, 1.35% and 1.2% of alkaloids, respectively, were mixed. What was the percentage strength of the mixture?

   _____

2. What is the percentage of alcohol in a mixture containing 150 ml of witch hazel (14% alcohol), 200 ml of glycerin, and 500 ml of 50% alcohol?

   _____

3. A pharmacy technician mixes 20 g of 10% ichthammol ointment, 45 g of 5% ichthammol ointment, and 100 g of petrolatum (diluent). What is the percentage of ichthammol in the finished compound?

   _____

   Rx   Coal Tar Solution (85% alcohol) 80 ml

   Glycerin   160 ml

   Alcohol (95% alcohol)   500 ml

   Boric Acid qs   1000 ml

   Sig: Use as a medicated lotion once a day.

4. Calculate the percentage of alcohol in the lotion.

   _____

5. A manufacturing pharmacy has four lots of ichthammol ointment, containing 50%, 25%, 10%, and 5% ichthammol. How many grams of each should be used in preparing 1 pound of 20% ichthammol ointment?

   _____

6. How much 95% and 30% alcohol should be mixed to make 1 pint of 70% alcohol?

   _____

7. How much 5% and 1% hydrocortisone should be mixed to make 1 pound of 2{½}% hydrocortisone ointment?

   _____

8. Prepare 1 liter of 0.75% sodium chloride solution from normal saline (0.9%) and {½} normal saline (0.45%). How much of each strength would be required to fill this order?

   _____

9. Prepare 1 liter of D-10-W using both D-5-W and D-20-W. How much of each strength would be required to fill this order?

   _____

10. Prepare 1 pound of 20% ointment using both 10% and 30% of the ointment. How much of each should be used?

    _____

Chapter **4** **Conversions and Calculations Used by Pharmacy Technicians**

IV Drip Rate Calculations

Objective: Calculate the drip (flow) rates, the number of drops per minute, or the amount of drug found in intravenous fluid administered to a patient.

Small-volume parenterals are injected into the body site slowly using a handheld syringe and needle. The medication is drawn into a syringe from a single dose ampule or a multidose vial. Some syringes are packaged prefilled by the manufacturer or hospital pharmacist or pharmacy technician.

Large-volume parenterals for continuous administration are hung at the patient's bed and are allowed to drip slowly into a vein by gravity flow or through the use of electrical or battery-operated volumetric infusion pumps. Some of these pumps can be calibrated to deliver "micro infusion" volumes such as 0.1 ml per hour or up to 2000 ml per hour, depending on the drug and requirements. Solutions of additive drugs are placed directly into large-volume parenterals or small-volume parenterals (minibags) containing the additive drug that may be hung piggyback and allowed to enter the tubing of the primary bottle of intravenous fluid and the patient at a controlled rate. In either situation, the physician specifies the rate of flow of intravenous fluids as milliliters per minute, as drops per minute of the amount of drug (milligrams, milliequivalents, or international units), or, more frequently, as the approximate duration of time of administration of the total volume.

In a hospital, the pharmacy is responsible for preparing fluids to be injected intravenously into a patient. The pharmacy technician may be required to calculate the flow or drip rate of an intravenous solution. The rate that a volume is infused can be calculated by using the following formula:

$$\frac{\text{Volume (milliliters)}}{\text{Time (hours)}}$$

At times, a pharmacy technician may be required to calculate the number of drops per minute that a patient is to receive. In this situation, the technician will need to know the flow rate and drop factor (number of drops per milliliter of the substance) and must use a conversion factor to convert hours to minutes. This can be done by using the following formula:

$$(\text{Drip or flow rate}) \, (\text{Drop factor}) \, (\text{Conversion factor}) = \text{Drop/min}$$

or

$$\frac{(\text{ml}) \times (\text{drops}) \times (1 \text{ hour})}{(\text{hour}) \times (\text{ml}) \times 60 \text{ minutes})} = \frac{\text{gtt}}{\text{minute}}$$

At other times, the pharmacy technician may need to calculate the amount of drug delivered over a specified period of time. This can be done by using the following formula:

$$\frac{\text{Amount of drug in IV bag}}{\text{Amount of drug delivered per unit of time}} = \frac{\text{Total volume of IV bag}}{\text{Volume delivered per unit of time}}$$

Lab Activity #4.9: Complete the following questions about IV drip rates.

Equipment needed:

- Calculator
- Pencil/pen
- Paper

Time needed to complete this activity: 30 minutes

1. 500 ml of a 2% sterile solution is to be administered by intravenous infusion over a period of 4 hours; how many milliliters will be administered over 1 hour?

   _____

2. A physician orders 1 liter of normal saline infused over 24 hours; how many milliliters of the intravenous solution will the patient receive after 8 hours?

   _____

3. What is the time of infusion of the drip (flow) rate?

_____

4. A physician prescribes 1 liter of D-20-W to be administered over 8 hours using an infusion kit with a drop factor of 10 gtt/ml. What will be the number of drops per minute?

_____

5. A physician writes a medication order for a patient of D-10-W q12h. The drop factor is set at 60 gtt/ml and the drip (flow) rate is 50 ml/hr. How many liters of fluid would be required to fill this order?

_____

6. A physician prescribes 1 liter of ½ NS to be infused at 6 ml/min and the drop factor is 20 gtt/ml. How many drops per minute will the patient receive?

_____

7. A physician prescribes 1000 ml of lactated Ringer's solution to be infused over 8 hours using a drop factor of 20 gtt/ml. How many gtt/min will the patient receive?

_____

8. A physician orders a 2-g vial of a drug to be added to 500 ml of D-5-W (5% dextrose in water for injection). If the administration rate is set at 125 ml per hour, how many milligrams of the drug will a patient receive per minute?

_____

9. A certain hyperalimentation fluid measures 1 liter. If the solution is to be administered over a period of hours and if the administration set is calibrated at 25 drops/ml, at what rate should the set be calibrated to administer the solution during the designated time interval?

_____

10. Five hundred (500) milliliters of an intravenous solution contains 0.2% of succinylcholine chloride in sodium chloride injection. At what rate should the infusion be administered to provide 2.5 mg of succinylcholine chloride per minute?

_____

Chapter **4** **Conversions and Calculations Used by Pharmacy Technicians**

5 Dosage Forms, Routes of Administration, and Drug Classifications, Drug Abbreviations, and Medical Terminology

TERMS AND DEFINITIONS

Select the correct term from the following list and write the corresponding letter in the blank next to the statement.

A. Absorption
B. Bioavailability
C. Bioequivalence
D. Distribution
E. Excretion
F. Half-life
G. Behind the counter (BTC)
H. Instill
I. Legend drugs
J. Over-the-counter (OTC)
K. Parenteral
L. Pharmacokinetics
M. Metabolism

___C___ 1. The relationship between two drugs that have the same dosage and dosage form with similar bioavailability

___F___ 2. The amount of time required for a chemical to be decreased by one half

___I___ 3. Drugs that require a prescription

___L___ 4. Life of the drug, which includes absorption, metabolism, distribution, and excretion

___K___ 5. Medication introduced other than by way of the intestines

___H___ 6. To place into; instructions used for ophthalmics or otics

___A___ 7. The ability of a drug to pass into the bloodstream or other target tissues

___D___ 8. Incorporation of a chemical agent across natural barriers of the body

___E___ 9. The process of elimination of medicinal agents

___G___ 10. Nonprescription drugs that are kept behind the pharmacy counter

___J___ 11. Medications that do not require a prescription

___B___ 12. Amount of drug that reaches intended destination by being absorbed into the bloodstream

___M___ 13. The process that breaks down drugs for excretion

TRUE OR FALSE

Write T or F next to each statement.

___T___ 1. To become proficient in the medical profession, a technician must be able to interpret orders correctly.

___T___ 2. Much of the terminology used in pharmacy comes from the Latin and Greek languages.

___F___ 3. It is not necessary for the pharmacy technician to learn all dosage forms and abbreviations to decipher a physician's orders.

___T___ 4. The number of errors resulting from physicians' poor handwriting or from transcription of orders is of little concern.

___T___ 5. The *dosage form* is the means by which a drug is available for use.

___T___ 6. An emulsion is a liquid dosage form.

___F___ 7. A troche is a semisolid dosage form.

_____T_____ 8. An emulsifier binds oil and water together in a mixture.

_____F_____ 9. Enemas used to treat constipation typically take longer than 10 hours to work.

_____T____10. Semisolid dosage forms are normally meant for topical applications.

_____T____11. Gels contain medication in a viscous thick liquid that easily penetrates the skin and does not leave a residue.

_____F____12. Lozenges are oral tablets that should be swallowed immediately.

_____T____13. Physicians frequently use eye solutions to treat ear conditions.

_____T____14. A patient's age, gender, genetics, and diet, as well as other chemicals in the body, can influence and alter metabolism.

_____T____15. If inhalers are not used properly, medication is swallowed rather than inhaled into the lungs.

MULTIPLE CHOICE

Complete each question by circling the best answer.

1. The directions for use of a medication are "ii gtts os bid." The route of administration is:
   A. Right eye
   B. Left eye
   C. Right ear
   D. Left ear

2. Which of the following is the abbreviation for "before meals"?
   A. ac
   B. pc
   C. hs
   D. au

3. The directions for use of a medication are "Tylenol 80 mg pr q6h prn." What dosage form should be dispensed?
   A. Chew tab
   B. Syrup
   C. Suppository
   D. Enema

4. The directions for use are "Nitrostat 1/200 gr sl prn." How should this be administered?
   A. In the left ear
   B. Very slowly
   C. Under the tongue
   D. Under the skin

5. When a drug is processed by the liver, this is referred to as:
   A. Absorption
   B. Distribution
   C. Metabolism
   D. Excretion

6. Which of the following dosage forms should generally be stored in the refrigerator?
   A. Suppositories
   B. Patches
   C. Enemas
   D. Tablets

7. Which route of administration has the quickest onset of action?
   A. IM
   B. PR
   C. IV
   D. PO

8. The directions for use are "I gtt od qd." The medication may be:
   A. Ear drops
   B. Eye drops
   C. Suppositories
   D. Vaginal tablets

9. The abbreviation *NGT* refers to:
   A. Nitroglycerin
   B. Nothing by gastrostomy tube
   C. Nasogastric
   D. Nasogastric tube

10. The pharmaceutical abbreviation *CD* refers to:
    A. Controlled drug
    B. Compact disk
    C. Controlled diffusion
    D. Continuous drip

11. A suspension should always have which auxiliary label?
    A. Keep refrigerated
    B. Shake well
    C. For external use only
    D. May cause drowsiness

12. Tablets are often identified by:
    A. Imprint codes
    B. Shape of tablet
    C. Color of tablet
    D. All of the above

13. A positive aspect of taking tablets, capsules, or any agent by mouth is:
    A. Convenience to the patient
    B. Physicians mainly write for those forms
    C. Injectable forms are expensive
    D. Medication can be taken with water

14. Respiratory solutions are often:
    A. Refrigerated
    B. Packaged in unit dose ampules
    C. For adult use only
    D. Purchased over-the-counter

15. Patients with diabetes may be instructed to buy drug products that are:
    A. Sugar-free
    B. Alcohol-free
    C. Both A and B
    D. None of the above

MATCHING

Match the following abbreviations with their meanings.

Matching I

E 1. Inh
H 2. PV
F 3. SubQ
A 4. IV
I 5. Top
J 6. IVPB
B 7. Inj
G 8. IM
D 9. PO
C 10. ID

A. Intravenous
B. Injectable
C. Intradermal
D. By mouth
E. Inhalant
F. Subcutaneous
G. Intramuscular
H. Vaginal
I. Topical
J. Intravenous piggyback

Matching II

G 1. tab
A 2. elix
H 3. lot
F 4. dil
J 5. cap
B 6. tinc
I 7. syr
D 8. ectab
E 9. ung
C 10. supp

A. Elixir
B. Tincture
C. Suppositories
D. Enteric-coated tablet
E. Ointment
F. Diluent
G. Tablet
H. Lotion
I. Syrup
J. Capsule

FILL IN THE BLANK

Answer each question by completing the statement in the space provided.

1. What type of tablet is best for children? _____

2. Three types of capsules are _____, _____, and _____.

3. What are two common uses for transdermal patches? _____ and _____
   _____.

4. Syrups are _____ based, and elixirs are _____ _____
   _____ based.

5. Suppositories may be administered _____ or _____.

6. The most commonly used SL tablet is _____.

7. Most topical agents work at the _____ _____ _____.

8. The last phase of a drug's life in the body is _____.

9. All types of dosage forms manufactured must be approved by the _____.

10. Name four types of semisolids: _____, _____, _____, and
    _____.

SHORT ANSWER

Write a short response to each question in the space provided.

1. Describe the "first-pass" effect of drugs in the liver.

   _____

   _____

   _____

2. How are medications packaged?

   _____

   _____

   _____

Follow the instructions given in each exercise and provide a response.

1. Visit a local pharmacy. Locate the cough and cold section. Select one brand of medication with the following dosage forms: tablet, capsule, and liquid. What are the active ingredients in all three dosage forms?

2. List as many dosage forms as you can. Write two advantages and two disadvantages of each.

   Example: Tablet—advantage, easy to carry; disadvantage, tastes bad

REFLECT CRITICALLY

CRITICAL THINKING

Reply to each question based on what you have learned in the chapter.

1. Interpreting prescriptions can be challenging because of the various handwriting styles of physicians. Think of three rules that can make this task easier.

   1- rule is a universal abbreviation system that all physicians agree to use.
   2- Dr verbally repeats/dictates order while writing to nurse present.
   3- Dr uses pre-printed sheet and just checkmarks boxes.

2. Five-year-old Tommy refuses to take his medication for iron deficiency anemia. The pharmacist has tried to mask the taste by using various compounds, but nothing seems to work. His mother finally asks for your help. What would you use that would make Tommy want to take his medicine?

   Pre dose w/ a tranquilizer/qualude to make him docile + obedient, then administer the medicine. Or make it into a patch that just sticks on skin. Or put it in a capsule to block taste.

3. Compounding medications unavailable commercially is much like creating a good recipe in the kitchen. Compare and contrast the two tasks. How are they similar, and how do they differ?

   Similar in that one is mixing several ingredients together to create a finished product. They differ in that the ingredients in compounding are probably far more expensive, and the ratios of ingredients must be extremely precise.

RELATE TO PRACTICE

LAB SCENARIOS

Medical Abbreviations

Objective: To introduce the pharmacy technician to the many abbreviations that may be encountered in the practice of pharmacy, regardless of the pharmacy setting.

Lab Activity #5.1: Write the meanings of the following medical abbreviations.

   Equipment needed:

   ▪ Pen/pencil

   Time needed to complete this activity: 20 minutes

Part 1

1. BM _____
2. BPH _____
3. CAD _____
4. COPD _____
5. DDS _____
6. HA _____
7. HBP _____
8. HTN _____
9. MD _____
10. OA _____
11. SLE _____
12. Dx _____
13. TB _____
14. TIA _____
15. UC _____
16. URI _____

Part 2

1. BP _____
2. BS _____
3. CHF _____
4. CP _____
5. DJD _____
6. GERD _____
7. UTI _____
8. GI _____
9. HR _____
10. PVCs _____
11. RA _____
12. SOB _____
13. Sx _____
14. TED _____
15. TX _____

Chapter **5** **Dosage Forms, Routes of Administration**

Medical Terminology

Objective: To become familiar with the meanings of prefixes, suffixes, and root words used in medical terminology.

Lab Activity #5.2: Interpreting the meanings of prefixes, suffixes, and root words that are found in medical literature associated with the practice of pharmacy.

Equipment needed:

- Medical terminology book
- Pencil/pen

Time needed to complete this activity: 60 minutes

Complete the following table of prefixes used in medical terminology.

Prefix	Meaning	Prefix	Meaning
a-; an-; ana-		micro-	
ab-		multi-	
ante-		neo-	
anti-		non-	
auto-		oligo-	
bi-		pan-	
brady-		para-	
carcin-		per-	
contra-		peri-	
dys-		poly-	
ect-		post-	
en-		pre-	
endo-		primi-	
epi-		retro-	
ex-		semi-	
gynec/o-		sub-	
hemi-		super-	
hyper-		supra-	
hypo-		sym-	
infra-		syn-	
inter-		tachy-	
intra-		tri-	
iso-		uni-	
macro-		xero-	
mal-			

Complete the following table of suffixes found in medical terminology.

Suffix	Meaning	Suffix	Meaning
-ac; -al;-ar; -ary		-paresis	
-algia		-pathy	
-cele		-penia	
-centesis		-pepsia	
-crine		-phagia	
-crit		-phobia	
-cyte		-phonia	
-cytosis		-phoresis	
-desis		-phoria	
-ectomy		-plasty	
-emesis		-plegia	
-emia		-pnea	
-genesis		-poiesis	
-globin; -globulin		-r/rhage;-r/rhagia	
-gram		-rrhea	
-graph		-rhexis	
-graphy		-sclerosis	
-ia; -iac;-ic		-scope	
-ism		-scopy	
-itis		-somnia	
-lysis;-lytic		-spasm	
-malacia		-stasis	
-megaly		-stenosis	
-oid		-therapy	
-(o)logist		-thorax	
-(o)logy		-tocia	
-oma		-tripsy	
-osis		-trophy	
-ostomy		-tropin	

Complete the following table of root words found in medical terminology.

Root Word	Meaning	Root Word	Meaning
abdomen/o		mast/o	
aden/o		melan/o	
adipo/o		men/o	
amino		metacarp/o	
andr/o		metatars/o	
angi/o		morph/.o	
aque/o		muc/o	
arteri/o		my/o	
arteriol/o		myc/o	
arthr/o		myel/o	
ather/o		miring/o	
audi/o		narc/o	
aur/o		nat/o	
bili		nephr/o	
blephar/o		neur/o	
bronch/o		noct/o	
bronchiol/o		nyctal/o	
bucc/o		ocul/o	
calc/i		onch/o	
capnia		oophor/o	
carcin/o		ophthalm/o	
cardi/o		opt/o	
carp/o		or/o	
cephal/o		orch/o	
cerebr/o		orchi/o	
chol/e		orchid/o	
cholangi/o		orth/o	
cholecyst/o		oste/o	
chondr/o		ot/o	
coagul/o		ovari/o	
cochle/o		oxi	
col/o		pachy/o	
conjunctiv/o		pancreat/o	
cor/o		par/o	
corne/o		part/o	
coron/o		patell/o	
cost/o		pector/o	
crani/o		ped	
cry/o		pelv/i	

Root Word	Meaning	Root Word	Meaning
cut/o		perine/o	
cutane/o		peritone/o	
cyan/o		phag/o	
cyst/o		phalang/o	
cyt/o		pharyng/o	
dacry/o		phleb/o	
dent		phot/o	
derm/o		phren/o	
dermat/o		pil/o	
dipi/o		pneum/o	
dipso/o		pod/o	
duoden/o		proct/o	
dur/a		psych/o	
electr/o		pub/o	
embry/o		pulmon/o	
encephal/o		py/o	
enter/o		pyel/o	
eosin/o		quadr/i	
epis/i		radi/o	
erythr/o		rect/o	
esophag/o		ren/o	
fasci/o		retin/o	
femor/o		rhabdomy/o	
fet/o		rheum	
fibul/o		rhin/o	
fund/o		salping/o	
gastr/o		sarc/o	
gingiv/o		semin/o	
glauc/o		septi	
gli/o		sial/o	
glomerul/o		sinus/o	
gloss/o		somat/o	
gluc/o		spermat/o	
glyc/o		spher/o	
gonad/o		sphygm/o	
gravid/a		spir/o	
gyn/o		splen/o	
gynec/o		spondyl/o	
hem/o		steth/o	
hemangi/o		stoma	

Continued

Root Word	Meaning	Root Word	Meaning
hemat/o		synovi/o	
hepat/o		tars/o	
hidr/o		ten/o	
humer/o		tendon/o	
hydr/o		test/o	
hyster/o		testicul/o	
ile/o		thorac/o	
ili/o		thromb/o	
immune/o		thyr/o	
is/o		trache/o	
jejun/o		tympan/o	
kal/i		ur/o	
kinesi/o		urethr/o	
lacrim/o		vas/o	
lact/o		ven/o	
lapar/o		xanth/o	
laryng/o		lil/o	
ligament/o		lumb/o	
lingua		mamm/o	

6 Drug Information References

TERMS AND DEFINITIONS

Select the correct term from the following list and write the corresponding letter in the blank next to the statement.

A. Chemical structure
B. Brand/trade name
C. Drug classification
D. Formulary
E. Generic name
F. Package insert
G. Non-formulary

_____ 1. A list of drugs not normally stocked by a pharmacy or not approved by drug coverage plan

_____ 2. A list of drugs approved for use from which choices are made

_____ 3. The shapes of molecules and their locations with regard to one another

_____ 4. Based on the action of a drug, its use, or its chemistry

_____ 5. Official prescribing information for a prescription drug

_____ 6. Trademark of a drug or device created by the original manufacturer

_____ 7. Nonproprietary name assigned to a medication by the manufacturer based on chemical characteristics

TRUE OR FALSE

Write T or F next to each statement.

_____ 1. Pharmacy reference books are used by pharmacy personnel only.

_____ 2. Pharmacists rely on drug information references to give correct information to health care workers.

_____ 3. Manufacturers give a drug a name based on its chemical attributes.

_____ 4. All brand, or trade, drug names should be capitalized.

_____ 5. Contraindications list the main conditions for which the drug is used.

_____ 6. All technicians should carry a *Facts and Comparisons* in their pocket.

_____ 7. Most generic drug names typically begin with J or W

_____ 8. Micromedex is one online drug information resource for pharmacy settings

_____ 9. *Physicians' Desk Reference* online subscription is free to patients

_____ 10. *United States Pharmacopeia-NF* provides access to official standards for quality control and manufacturing of drugs

MULTIPLE CHOICE

Complete each question by circling the best answer.

1. A reference text familiar to most pharmacists is:
   A. *Facts and Comparisons*
   B. *Physicians' Desk Reference*
   C. *The Red Book*
   D. *United States Pharmacopeia*

2. The section of *Facts and Comparisons* that shows in color 250 of the most frequently used drugs is:
   A. Index
   B. Drug monograph
   C. Drug identification
   D. Appendix

3. The reference book known as the *PDR* is the:
   A. *Pharmacists' Drug Reference*
   B. *Physicians' Desk Reference*
   C. *Pharmacist Desk Reference*
   D. *Pharmacy Dosage Regulations*

4. The PDR contains what information?
   A. Manufacturers' addresses and phone numbers
   B. Manufacturer-provided package inserts for select FDA-approved drugs
   C. Products listed by classification or method of action
   D. All of the above

5. The diagnostic product information section of the PDR contains:
   A. A key to controlled substances
   B. A key to FDA pregnancy ratings
   C. An FDA telephone directory
   D. Information on drug products used as diagnostic agents

6. If a technician must know the upper limit price and rules or the billing units for each type of drug under state AIDS drug assistance programs, he/she would use:
   A. *Facts and Comparisons*
   B. *Physicians' Desk Reference*
   C. *The Red Book*
   D. *Orange Book Code*

7. A patient has taken a drug in tablet form but does not know what it is; the technician might use which reference to find out what the drug is?
   A. *American Hospital Formulary Service Drug Information*
   B. *United States Pharmacopeia Drug Information*
   C. *Ident-A-Drug*
   D. *The Injectable Drug Handbook*

8. The book used to reference the compatibility of various parenteral agents is:
   A. *American Hospital Formulary Service Drug Information*
   B. *United States Pharmacopeia Drug Information*
   C. *Ident-A-Drug*
   D. *The Injectable Drug Handbook*

9. *Facts and Comparisons* in book form is updated:
   A. Monthly
   B. Yearly
   C. A and B
   D. None of the above

10. Pharmacy journals contain information about:
    A. New drugs
    B. The future of pharmacy
    C. Legislative changes
    D. All of the above

11. Currently, only one association is run by technicians and allows only pharmacy technicians as members. It is the:
    A. NPTA
    B. AAPT
    C. ASHP
    D. APhA

12. Of the sources listed here, which would be best for finding a recommendation for a sugar-free and alcohol-free cough syrup?
    A. *Physicians' Desk Reference*
    B. *Red Book*
    C. *Facts and Comparisons*
    D. *Ident-A-Drug*

13. *Clinical Pharmacology* is an electronic drug compendium used in:
    A. Retail pharmacies
    B. Hospital pharmacies
    C. Physicians' offices
    D. All of the above

14. *Clinical Xpert* provides online and mobile applications used by:
    A. Pharmacists and technicians
    B. Physicians and nurses
    C. Both A and B
    D. None of the above

15. _____ offers basic free drug information that can be downloaded onto a personal computer or handheld device.
    A. *Epocrates*
    B. *Remington's Pharmaceutical Sciences*
    C. *American Drug Index*
    D. *Red Book*

MATCHING

Match the following abbreviations with their meanings.

Matching I

_____ 1. FDA

_____ 2. Monographs

_____ 3. Contraindications

_____ 4. Indications

_____ 5. Classification

A. Package inserts
B. Identifies the types of people who should not be given a drug
C. Approves all new drugs
D. Categorizes drugs based on chemistry, actions, or uses
E. Lists main conditions for which a chemical is used

Matching II

_____ 1. UPC

_____ 2. AWP

_____ 3. NDC

_____ 4. USP

_____ 5. F&C

A. Average wholesale price
B. *Facts and Comparisons*
C. *United States Pharmacopeia*
D. Universal Product Code
E. National Drug Code

FILL IN THE BLANK

Answer each question by completing the statement in the space provided.

1. _____ _____ _____ is a reference commonly used in pharmacies.

2. The reference text most often used in a physician's office is the _____.

3. The _____ book is a good source of information on drug costs.

4. The _____ book is a comprehensive listing of approved drug products with therapeutic equivalent evaluations.

5. A comprehensive listing of prescription drugs and their uses, precautions, and adverse reactions that is used primarily in the hospital is the _____.

6. Pharmacy organizations have _____ on the Internet.

7. _____ should not be limited to books alone.

8. Many websites provide _____ _____ in the form of _____

   _____ and _____ _____ _____.

9. Another way to attain new drug information is to join an _____.

10. All _____ _____ _____ never stop acquiring information.

RESEARCH ACTIVITY

Follow the instructions given in each exercise and provide a response.

1. Access the websites listed in Table 6-6 of the textbook. Describe the type of information provided on each website.

REFLECT CRITICALLY

CRITICAL THINKING

Reply to each question based on what you have learned in the chapter.

1. Of all the reference books discussed in this chapter, which one seems to be the easiest to use and understand?

2. Think of some of the magazines you have read or glanced through lately at a newsstand. How many of them included some sort of medical, drug, or health-related article or information? Did the articles spark your interest? If so, why? Were any of them written by professionals in the field?

3. List as many sources as possible that could be used as resources for drug information and that can be accessed without the need to buy a book on the subject.

RELATE TO PRACTICE

LAB SCENARIOS

Reference Materials

Objective: To familiarize the pharmacy technician with various forms of reference materials and the terminology associated with each.

Each pharmacy regardless of the setting is required by state boards of pharmacy to maintain a library relevant to its practice. State boards of pharmacy require that a pharmacy maintain a current edition of the *USP-NF* (the official compendium in the United States) and a copy of the United States Controlled Substance Act.

A pharmacy technician must be familiar with proper usage of these reference materials, which may consist of books, journals, and pharmacy magazines. In many situations, these materials may be found in an electronic format.

Lab Activity #6.1: Use the *Physicians' Desk Reference (PDR)* or *Drug Facts and Comparisons* to define the terms found in these reference materials.

Equipment needed:

- *Physicians' Desk Reference* (PDR) or *Drug Facts and Comparisons*
- Pencil/pen

Time needed to complete this activity: 15 minutes

Define the following terms used in pharmacy reference materials.

1. Adverse reactions

   _____

2. Clinical pharmacology

   _____

3. Contraindication

   _____

4. Description

   _____

5. Dosage and administration

   _____

6. How supplied

   _____

7. Indication

   _____

8. Mechanism of action

   _____

9. Monograph

   _____

10. Pharmacokinetics

    _____

11. Precautions

    _____

12. Teratogenic effects

    _____

13. Warnings

    _____

Lab Activity #6.2: Use *Approved Drug Products with Therapeutic Equivalence Evaluations (Orange Book)* to define the following terms found in drug monographs.

Equipment needed:

- Computer with Internet connection *(www.fda.gov)*
- Pencil/pen

Time needed to complete this activity: 10 minutes

Define the following terms.

1. Pharmaceutical equivalents

_____

2. Pharmaceutical alternatives

_____

3. Therapeutic equivalent

_____

4. Bioavailability

_____

5. Bioequivalent drug products

_____

Lab Activity #6.3: Use *Approved Drug Products with Therapeutic Equivalence Evaluations (Orange Book)* to define the following therapeutic equivalent evaluation codes.

Equipment needed:

- Computer with Internet connection *(www.fda.gov)* to access *Approved Drug Products with Therapeutic Evaluations (Orange Book)*
- Pencil/pen

Time needed to complete this activity: 15 minutes

Define the following therapeutic equivalent evaluation codes.

1. A

_____

2. AA

_____

3. AB

_____

4. AN

_____

5. AO

_____

6. AP

_____

7. AT

_____

8. B

_____

9. BC

_____

10. BD

_____

11. BE

_____

12. BN

_____

13. BP

_____

14. BR

_____

15. BS

_____

16. BT

_____

17. BX

_____

7 Prescription Processing

TERMS AND DEFINITIONS

Select the correct term from the following list and write the corresponding letter in the blank next to the statement.

A. Auxiliary label
B. Automated dispensing system
C. Closed door pharmacy
D. E-prescribing
E. Institutional pharmacy
F. Community pharmacy
G. Digital counters
H. Rx
I. Script
J. Sig

_G_ 1. Counts tablets or capsules as they are poured into the vials

_I_ 2. Another name for a prescription

_B_ 3. Computerized automated machines that hold a supply of various medications

_E_ 4. Pharmacy in a hospital setting, may or may not provide retail services

_D_ 5. Electronically sent prescription from a computer or mobile device

_C_ 6. Not open to the public, services long-term care facilities or mail order pharmacies

_H_ 7. Latin abbreviation for "recipe"; commonly used to mean "prescription"

_F_ 8. Written prescriptions usually hand carried by a patient to be filled in this setting

_A_ 9. Attached to a container with specific instructions or information pertaining to the medication inside

_J_ 10. Medication directions written in pharmacy terms on a prescription

TRUE OR FALSE

Write T or F next to each statement.

_T_ 1. One of the most important duties performed by a technician is filling prescriptions.

_F_ 2. If technicians cannot interpret the information on a prescription, they should quickly make an educated guess.

_F_ 3. Five basic steps are involved in filling a prescription, and all five relate directly to the technician.

_T_ 4. The person at the take-in counter is usually the first one to handle the script in the pharmacy.

_F_ 5. If a prescription is filled by a technician incorrectly, the outcome affects only the technician who filled the order.

_F_ 6. Most court cases favor the pharmacist and award the pharmacy cash settlements.

_F_ 7. All vials leaving the pharmacy must, by law, have childproof lids—no exceptions.

_T_ 8. The technician should check the medication against the script and the label when selecting medication from the shelf.

_T_ 9. The prescription label must show the name, address, and phone number of the pharmacy.

_T_ 10. The last step in filling prescriptions is to pass the prescription to the pharmacist for final inspection and signature.

Complete the question by circling the best answer.

1. When taking in a prescription, neither the technician nor the pharmacist can decipher the physician's writing; therefore:
   A. The technician should guess what to fill
   B. The technician should ask the patient
   C. The pharmacist should call the physician
   D. The technician should tell the patient to go back to the doctor and get a prescription that can be read

2. Which of the following is *not* the duty of a technician upon taking in a prescription?
   A. Translating the prescription
   B. Entering information into the database
   C. Filling the prescription
   D. Providing patient consultation

3. When a new prescription is called in to the pharmacy, who can take the prescription over the phone?
   A. Pharmacy clerk
   B. Pharmacy technician
   C. Pharmacist
   D. Pharmacy custodian

4. If a prescription is for a controlled substance, the technician must make sure the prescription includes the physician's:
   A. FDA number
   B. DEA number
   C. HMO number
   D. NABP number

5. Most dosing in an inpatient pharmacy is set in the medication cart for a _____ period.
   A. 12-hour
   B. 24-hour
   C. 36-hour
   D. 48-hour

6. Which of the following is *not* an exception to the safety lid law?
   A. Nitroglycerin
   B. Patient's request
   C. Isosorbide SL
   D. Technician's opinion that the patient looks too weak to open a safety lid

7. Which of the following is *not* preprinted on a prescription label as required by law?
   A. Name, address, and phone number of prescriber
   B. Prescription number
   C. Drug, strength, and dosage form
   D. Refill information

8. Which of the following is *not* a common auxiliary label for opioids?
   A. May cause drowsiness/dizziness
   B. May cause sensitivity to light
   C. Do not drink alcohol
   D. Alcohol may increase the effects of the drug

9. Which of the following is *not* an advantage of computer-dispensing systems?
   A. They have a high cost
   B. They increase productivity
   C. They cut down on errors
   D. They allow for better inventory control

10. The law states that all prescriptions must be kept on file for at least
    A. 6 months
    B. 1 year
    C. 2 years
    D. 5 years

11. Prescriptions that have a red "C" stamped on the right side when filed in the pharmacy indicate that the prescription is:
    A. A controlled substance
    B. A cough medication
    C. A drug containing codeine
    D. A cardiac medication

12. Pharmacy technicians must be capable of:
    A. Interpreting and transcribing prescriptions
    B. Filling prescriptions quickly and accurately
    C. Following proper billing practices
    D. All of the above

13. According to federal law, when should a patient receive counseling?
    A. At the last refill of the patient's medication
    B. Only when the patient asks for it
    C. When a new prescription is filled
    D. At all times

14. Most boards of pharmacy prefer to allow transfer of prescriptions only _____ time(s).
    A. One
    B. Two
    C. Three
    D. Zero

15. If the medication has to be counted or measured:
    A. Have the pharmacist check measurements
    B. Put medication into a bottle of appropriate size
    C. Place into the refrigerator
    D. None of the above

Write a short response to each question in the space provided.

1. List the five rights of the patient to medication safety.

   A. _____

   B. _____

   C. _____

   D. _____

   E. _____

2. List the five steps of processing a prescription.

   A. _____

   B. _____

   C. _____

   D. _____

   E. _____

3. What should be checked before a prescription is released to a relative?

   A. _____

   B. _____

4. What are the "meat and potatoes" of pharmacy? _____

   _____

   _____

5. List some examples of inpatient and outpatient dispensing systems. _____

   _____

   _____

6. When you check the label against the script, for what are you checking? _____

   _____

   _____

7. Why is it that many elderly patients do not want safety lids on their medications? _____

   _____

   _____

8. Why should technicians initial any prescriptions that they fill? _____

_____

_____

9. Many computer systems have a labeling system. What information is printed on one sheet?

_____

_____

10. When labeling prescription bottles a technician should remember professionalism; why is this important?

_____

_____

_____

RESEARCH ACTIVITY

Follow the instructions given in each exercise and provide a response. Access the websites www.carefusion.com *and* www.mckesson.com.

1. Look up news and events. What are the latest automated technology/products in development for pharmacies?

2. How many different products for automation are there?

REFLECT CRITICALLY

CRITICAL THINKING

Reply to each question based on what you have learned in the chapter.

1. Give five differences between outpatient and inpatient settings in handling of prescriptions/medication orders.

   1- Inpatient may not be open to public
   2- Physician with has much more presence
   3- Inpatient usually fills for 24 hr period
   4- Address of prescriber not necessary inpatient
   5- Inpatient higher salary!

Chapter **7** **Prescription Processing**

2. You have received a medication order for a chemotherapy drug in the pharmacy. You are the technician preparing chemotherapy when the order comes in by fax. You are not sure what the drug is on the order, so you consult the pharmacist. After some discussion, the two of you decide what the drug is, and the order is prepared. Who else would be able to verify that this is the correct medication before it is administered to the patient?

The Physician whose name/number should be on the fax

3. After filling about 25 prescriptions on a very busy morning in the pharmacy, you realize that you might have made a mistake on the last one. It is time to go to lunch, so you decide to let it go, believing that the pharmacist will catch it. Unfortunately, the pharmacist checks the prescription hurriedly, trusting that you did your job correctly, and the prescription goes home with the patient.

A. What should you have done to prevent this medication error?

Triple checked your work and told the pharmacist on your lunch about your error. Never assume your mistakes will be caught

B. Whose fault is it that the prescription was dispensed as is?

Yours and the pharmacist's.

C. What can you do to remedy the situation before the patient is harmed by your mistake?

Call patient, if no answer ask pharmacist but may be necessary to go to patient's house

RELATE TO PRACTICE

LAB SCENARIOS

The Prescription
Objective: To familiarize the pharmacy technician with the information required in a legal prescription.

Every day, retail pharmacies receive prescriptions for patients. A prescription is an order for a specific medication prescribed by a physician or other health care professional such as a physician assistant or a nurse practitioner, who is permitted by state law to prescribe medications. Each prescription must contain specific information if the pharmacy is to fill the order.

Information required on a prescription includes the following:
- Prescriber information: name, office address, office telephone number, NPI number, and DEA number if the prescription is a controlled substance
- Patient information: patient's name, birth date, and home address. A pharmacy will attempt to obtain a telephone number for the patient
- Date: the date on which the prescription was written. This date may be different from the date the prescription is filled
- Rx symbol: a symbol for a Latin word meaning "recipe" or "take this drug"
- Inscription: medication prescribed, which may be listed under the brand or generic name, and the strength and quantity of the drug to be dispensed
- Subscription: instructions to the pharmacist on dispensing the medication
- Signa (sig): directions for the patient to follow
- Additional filling information, such as refills permitted or generic substitution
- Prescriber's signature

Lab Activity #7.1: Identify what is missing from the following prescriptions.

Equipment needed:

- Pen/pencil

Time needed to complete this activity: 15 minutes

1. Rx 1:

```
                        Dr. Andrew A. Sheen
                   1100 Brentwood Blvd, Suite M780
                        St. Louis, MO 63144
                           314-527-0000
                          DEA FS1234563

   Brian Waters                                    January 12, 201X


   Rx      Amoxicillin 500 mg   #30
           1 cap po tid

   Ref x 1                          Dr. Andrew Sheen
```

What is missing on this prescription?

_____

2. Rx 2:

```
                        Dr. Andrew A. Sheen
                   1100 Brentwood Blvd, Suite M780
                        St. Louis, MO 63144
                           314-527-0000
                          DEA FS1234563

   Brian Waters                                    January 12, 201X
   4433 Simon Blvd, Apt 321, St. Louis, MO 63144

   Rx      Naprosyn 375 mg    #30
           1 tab po tid prn back pain

   Ref x 2
```

What is missing on this prescription?

_____

3. Rx 3:

```
                        Dr. Andrew A. Sheen
                   1100 Brentwood Blvd, Suite M780
                        St. Louis, MO 63144
                           314-527-0000
                          DEA FS1234563

   Brian Waters
   4433 Simon Blvd, Apt 321, St. Louis, MO 63144

   Rx     Z-pak  #6
          2 caps po stat, then I cap po qd x 4 days

   Ref x 1                          Dr. Andrew Sheen
```

What is missing on this prescription?

_____

4. Rx 4:

```
                    Dr. Andrew A. Sheen
                1100 Brentwood Blvd, Suite M780
                    St. Louis, MO 63144
                       314-527-0000
                     DEA FS1234563

Brian Waters                              January 12, 201X
4433 Simon Blvd, Apt 321, St. Louis, MO 63144

Rx      Lotrisone Cream
        Apply to the affected rash on arm twice a day

Ref x 1                         Dr. Andrew Sheen
```

What is missing on this prescription?

_____

5. Rx 5:

```
                    Dr. Andrew A. Sheen
                1100 Brentwood Blvd, Suite M780
                    St. Louis, MO 63144
                       314-527-0000
                       703-527-0000
Brian Waters                              January 12, 201X
4433 Simon Blvd, Apt 321, St. Louis, MO 63144

Rx      Vicodin      #30
        1 tab po tid prn pain

Ref x 1                         Dr. Andrew Sheen
```

What is missing on this prescription?

_____

6. Rx 6:

```
                    Dr. Andrew A. Sheen
                1100 Brentwood Blvd, Suite M780
                    St. Louis, MO 63144
                       314-527-0000
                     DEA FS1234563

Brian Waters                              January 12, 201X
4433 Simon Blvd, Apt 321, St. Louis, MO 63144

Rx      Flexeril     #30
        1 tab po tid prn muscle spasms

Ref x 1                         Dr. Andrew Sheen
```

What is missing on this prescription?

_____

7. Rx 7:

> Dr. Andrew A. Sheen
> 1100 Brentwood Blvd, Suite M780
> St. Louis, MO 63144
> 314-527-0000
> DEA FS1234563
>
> Brian Waters   January 12, 201X
> 4433 Simon Blvd, Apt 321, St. Louis, MO 63144
>
> Rx   Xalantan eye drops   1 bottle
>   UD
>
> Ref x 1   Dr. Andrew Sheen

What is missing on this prescription?

_____

8. Rx 8:

> Dr. Andrew A. Sheen
> 1100 Brentwood Blvd, Suite M780
> St. Louis, MO 63144
> 314-527-0000
> DEA FS1234563
> Brian Waters   January 12, 201X
> 4433 Simon Blvd, Apt 321, St. Louis, MO 63144
>
> Rx   Synthroid 0.15 mg   #30
>   1 tab po qd
>
> Ref x 6   Dr. Andrew Sheen

What is missing on this prescription?

_____

9. Rx 9:

> Dr. Andrew A. Sheen
> 1100 Brentwood Blvd, Suite M780
> St. Louis, MO 63144
> 314-527-0000
> DEA FS1234563
>
>   January 12, 201X
> 4433 Simon Blvd, Apt 321, St. Louis, MO 63144
>
> Rx   Xanax 0.5 mg   #60
>   1 tab po tid prn anxiety
>
> Ref x 5   Dr. Andrew Sheen

What is missing on this prescription?

_____

10. Rx 10:

```
                    Dr. Andrew A. Sheen
                 1100 Brentwood Blvd, Suite M780
                     St. Louis, MO 63144
                        314-527-0000
                       DEA FS1234563

Brian Waters                                          January 12, 201X
4433 Simon Blvd, Apt 321, St. Louis, MO 63144

Rx      Coreg
        1 tab po tid

Ref x 1                                    Dr. Andrew Sheen
```

What is missing on this prescription?

_____

Lab Activity #7.2: View the following DEA numbers and determine whether each is valid. If a number is not a valid DEA number, explain why.

Equipment needed:

- Pencil/pen
- Calculator

Time needed to complete this activity: 5 minutes

1. Dr. Andrew Sheen   AS123987

_____

2. Dr. William Dagit   BD7643219

_____

3. Dr. Jerry Kraisinger   JK1234563

_____

4. Dr. Richard Kunze   RK5555555

_____

5. Dr. Bruce Fisher   BF1236578

_____

6. Dr. Clark Andersen   FD4596328

_____

Interpreting a Prescription

Objective: To properly identify the specific information that must be entered into a pharmacy's computer for processing and reimbursement for the prescription.

In a community pharmacy setting, the pharmacy technician may be asked to enter the information from the prescription into the pharmacy's computer (information) system. The computer system prompts the technician to enter information in a particular sequence. Although each organization's system is unique, the information requested is the same.

The technician will be asked to enter the quantity of the medication being dispensed in metric terms, such as the number of tablets or capsules. If an ointment or cream is prescribed, it will be dispensed in grams, and if a liquid is prescribed, it will be dispensed in milliliters.

The day's supply can be calculated by dividing the quantity dispensed by the total amount taken during the day. The prescriber must indicate the number of refills permitted on the prescription. If no refills are indicated, the technician would indicate "0." Some physicians may indicate "prn" refills on a prescription. Depending on state board of pharmacy regulations, most states will permit a "prn" refill to be valid for 1 year from the date the prescription is written.

The pharmacy technician will be required to select the appropriate DAW code. Before selecting the DAW code, the pharmacy technician must determine whether the prescriber will permit a generic drug to be dispensed. A pharmacy will dispense a generic medication unless the physician writes in his/her own handwriting one of the following: "Brand Name Medically Necessary," "Dispense as Written," or "DAW." Most state boards of pharmacy no longer recognize the checking of boxes to indicate whether a generic can be dispensed. If in doubt, refer to your state board of pharmacy's regulations involving generic substitution.

The following are approved DAW codes:

DAW 0: no product selection indicated
DAW 1: substitution not allowed by provider
DAW 2: substitution allowed: patient-requested product dispensed
DAW 3: substitution allowed: pharmacist-selected product dispensed
DAW 4: substitution allowed: generic drug not in stock
DAW 5: substitution allowed: brand drug dispensed as generic
DAW 6: override
DAW 7: substitution not allowed: brand drug mandated by law
DAW 8: substitution allowed: generic drug not available in marketplace
DAW 9: other

If a pharmacy technician selects the incorrect DAW code, the pharmacy may not be properly reimbursed by a third-party provider.

Lab Activity #7.3: Answer the questions based on the prescription orders for each question.

Equipment needed:

- *Physicians' Desk Reference* or *Drug Facts and Comparisons*
- Pen/pencil
- Calculator

Time needed to complete this activity: 45 minutes

1. Rx 1:

   Augmentin 250 mg #30

   1 tab PO tid c̄ yogurt

   Ref ×1

a. How much will be dispensed (use metric quantities)?

_____

b. How many days will the medication last?

_____

c. How many refills are permitted on the prescription?

_____

d. What DAW code will be used?

_____

e. Write the directions as they would appear on the medication label.

_____

_____

_____

f. What auxiliary label(s) should be affixed to the medication label?

_____

_____

2. Rx 2:

Ampicillin 250 mg/tsp 200 ml

1 tsp PO qid ac and hs

Ref ×2

a. How much will be dispensed (use metric quantities)?

_____

b. How many days will the medication last?

_____

c. How many refills are permitted on the prescription?

_____

d. What DAW code will be used?

_____

e. Write the directions as they would appear on the medication label.

_____

_____

_____

f. What auxiliary label(s) should be affixed to the medication label?

_____

_____

3. Rx 3:

Zithromax 250 mg #6

2 caps PO stat, then 1 cap qd × 4 days

a. How much will be dispensed (use metric quantities)?

_____

b. How many days will the medication last?

_____

c. How many refills are permitted on the prescription?

_____

d. What DAW code will be used?

_____

e. Write the directions as they would appear on the medication label.

_____

_____

_____

f. What auxiliary label(s) should be affixed to the medication label?

_____

_____

_____

4. Rx 4:

Cortisporin Otic Soln 7.5 ml

gtts V in left ear q6h

Ref ×2

a. How much will be dispensed (use metric quantities)?

_____

b. How many days will the medication last?

_____

c. How many refills are permitted on the prescription?

_____

d. What DAW code will be used?

_____

e. Write the directions as they would appear on the medication label.

_____

_____

_____

f. What auxiliary label(s) should be affixed to the medication label?

_____

_____

5. Rx 5:

Doxycycline 100 mg 1 month supply

1 cap PO qd

Ref ×6

a. How much will be dispensed (use metric quantities)?

_____

b. How many days will the medication last?

_____

c. How many refills are permitted on the prescription?

_____

d. What DAW code will be used?

_____

e. Write the directions as they would appear on the medication label.

_____

_____

_____

f. What auxiliary label(s) should be affixed to the medication label?

_____

_____

_____

6. Rx 6:

Tylenol #3 #30 (Hint: Controlled Substance Schedule III)

1-2 tab PO q4-6h prn pain

Ref ×ii

a. How much will be dispensed (use metric quantities)?

_____

b. How many days will the medication last?

_____

c. How many refills are permitted on the prescription?

_____

d. What DAW code will be used?

_____

e. Write the directions as they would appear on the medication label.

_____

_____

_____

f. What auxiliary label(s) should be affixed to the medication label?

_____

_____

7. Rx 7:

   Flonase Nasal Spray 14.2 ml (120 sprays)
   2 spr to each nost bid
   Ref ×6

a. How much will be dispensed (use metric quantities)?

_____

b. How many days will the medication last?

_____

c. How many refills are permitted on the prescription?

_____

d. What DAW code will be used?

_____

e. Write the directions as they would appear on the medication label.

_____

_____

_____

f. What auxiliary label(s) should be affixed to the medication label?

_____

_____

8. Rx 8:

Viscous Xylocaine 100 ml

1 tsp PO swish and spit qid

a. How much will be dispensed (use metric quantities)?

_____

b. How many days will the medication last?

_____

c. How many refills are permitted on the prescription?

_____

d. What DAW code will be used?

_____

e. Write the directions as they would appear on the medication label.

_____

_____

_____

f. What auxiliary label(s) should be affixed to the medication label?

_____

_____

9. Rx 9:

Naprosyn 375 mg #30

1 tab PO tid c food

a. How much will be dispensed (use metric quantities)?

_____

b. How many days will the medication last?

_____

c. How many refills are permitted on the prescription?

_____

d. What DAW code will be used?

_____

e. Write the directions as they would appear on the medication label.

_____

_____

_____

f. What auxiliary label(s) should be affixed to the medication label?

_____

_____

10. Rx 10:

Prednisone 5 mg

ii tab PO qd × 5 d; i tab qd × 5d. Take with milk.

Ref

a. How much will be dispensed (use metric quantities)?

_____

b. How many days will the medication last?

_____

c. How many refills are permitted on the prescription?

_____

d. What DAW code will be used?

_____

e. Write the directions as they would appear on the medication label.

_____

_____

_____

f. What auxiliary label(s) should be affixed to the medication label?

_____

_____

11. Rx 11:

Terazol 3 Vag supp 1 box of 3

1 supp pv q hs

Ref ×1

a. How much will be dispensed (use metric quantities)?

_____

b. How many days will the medication last?

_____

c. How many refills are permitted on the prescription?

_____

d. What DAW code will be used?

_____

e. Write the directions as they would appear on the medication label.

_____

_____

_____

f. What auxiliary label(s) should be affixed to the medication label?

_____

_____

12. Rx 12:

Sporanox 200 mg #7

1 cap PO qd c̄ food for 7 d, skip 21 d and resume

Ref ×6

a. How much will be dispensed (use metric quantities)?

_____

b. How many days will the medication last?

_____

c. How many refills are permitted on the prescription?

_____

d. What DAW code will be used?

_____

e. Write the directions as they would appear on the medication label.

_____

_____

_____

f. What auxiliary label(s) should be affixed to the medication label?

_____

_____

13. Rx 13:

Flagyl 250 mg 14 day supply

1 tab PO qid for patient for 14 days. No alcohol.

Brand Name Medically Necessary

a. How much will be dispensed (use metric quantities)?

_____

b. How many days will the medication last?

_____

c. How many refills are permitted on the prescription?

_____

d. What DAW code will be used?

_____

e. Write the directions as they would appear on the medication label.

_____

_____

_____

f. What auxiliary label(s) should be affixed to the medication label?

_____

_____

14. Rx 14:

Proventil HFA Inhaler (200 sprays) #ii inhalers

1-2 inhalations in each nos q4-6h prn asthma and 15 min before exercise

Ref ×6

a. How much will be dispensed (use metric quantities)?

_____

b. How many days will the medication last?

_____

c. How many refills are permitted on the prescription?

_____

d. What DAW code will be used?

_____

e. Write the directions as they would appear on the medication label.

_____

_____

_____

f. What auxiliary label(s) should be affixed to the medication label?

_____

_____

15. Rx 15:

Coumadin 5 mg #45

1 tab PO odd numbered days, 2 tab PO even numbered days

DAW

Ref prn

a. How much will be dispensed (use metric quantities)?

_____

b. How many days will the medication last?

_____

c. How many refills are permitted on the prescription?

_____

d. What DAW code will be used?

_____

e. Write the directions as they would appear on the medication label.

_____

_____

_____

f. What auxiliary label(s) should be affixed to the medication label?

_____

_____

16. Rx 16:

Dilantin 100 mg #120

1 cap PO qid ac and hs

Dispense as Written

Ref ×6

a. How much will be dispensed (use metric quantities)?

_____

b. How many days will the medication last?

_____

c. How many refills are permitted on the prescription?

_____

d. What DAW code will be used?

_____

e. Write the directions as they would appear on the medication label.

_____

_____

_____

f. What auxiliary label(s) should be affixed to the medication label?

_____

_____

17. Rx 17:

Synthroid 0.1 mg #30

1 tab PO qd

Brand Name Medically Necessary

Ref ×3

a. How much will be dispensed (use metric quantities)?

_____

b. How many days will the medication last?

_____

c. How many refills are permitted on the prescription?

_____

d. What DAW code will be used?

_____

e. Write the directions as they would appear on the medication label.

_____

_____

_____

f. What auxiliary label(s) should be affixed to the medication label?

_____

_____

18. Rx 18:

Zoloft 100 mg #30

1 tab PO q am

Ref ×3

a. How much will be dispensed (use metric quantities)?

_____

b. How many days will the medication last?

_____

c. How many refills are permitted on the prescription?

_____

d. What DAW code will be used?

_____

e. Write the directions as they would appear on the medication label.

_____

_____

_____

f. What auxiliary label(s) should be affixed to the medication label?

_____

_____

19. Rx 19:

Zovirax 200 mg #25

1 cap PO q4h (5 times per day)

Ref ×2

a. How much will be dispensed (use metric quantities)?

_____

b. How many days will the medication last?

_____

c. How many refills are permitted on the prescription?

_____

d. What DAW code will be used?

_____

e. Write the directions as they would appear on the medication label.

_____

_____

_____

f. What auxiliary label(s) should be affixed to the medication label?

_____

_____

20. Rx 20:

Cephulac Syrup 1 pint

1 tbsp PO bid prn constipation

Ref ×6

a. How much will be dispensed (use metric quantities)?

_____

b. How many days will the medication last?

_____

c. How many refills are permitted on the prescription?

_____

d. What DAW code will be used?

_____

e. Write the directions as they would appear on the medication label.

_____

_____

f. What auxiliary labels should be affixed to the medication label?

_____

Reviewing the Prescription

Objective: To demonstrate the importance of multiple checks during the prescription filling process.

> During the prescription filling process, a pharmacy technician should check the prescription at least three times.

Lab Activity #7.4: Identify the error that appears on the prescription label.

Equipment needed:

- Pen/pencil
- List of pharmacy abbreviations

Time needed to complete this activity: 15 minutes

1. Rx 1:

```
                        Dr. Andrew A. Sheen
                    1100 Brentwood Blvd, Suite M780
                         St. Louis, MO 63144
                            314-527-0000
                           DEA FS1234563

Brian Waters                                       January 12, 201X
4433 Simon Blvd, Apt 321, St. Louis, MO 63144
DOB 12/2/1956

Rx      Amoxicillin    500 mg             #30
           1 cap po tid

Ref x 1                              Dr. Andrew Sheen
```

Prescription label:

```
                    Your Friendly Pharmacy
                       1234 Park Avenue
                      Arlington, VA 22209
                  703-243-0036; Fax 703-243-0037

Rx 1001                        Date 1/13/201X
Brian Waters                   Dr. Shedlock
DOB:  12/2/1956

4433 Simon Blvd, Apt 321, St. Louis, MO 63144
Amoxicillin 500 mg                      #30
Take one capsule by mouth four times a day.
Refills: 1
```

Identify the error on the prescription label and indicate how it should be corrected.

_____

_____

_____

2. Rx 2:

```
                    Dr. Andrew A. Sheen
                1100 Brentwood Blvd, Suite M780
                    St. Louis, MO 63144
                       314-527-0000
                      DEA FS1234563

Brian Waters                                    January 12, 201X
4433 Simon Blvd, Apt 321, St. Louis, MO 63144
DOB: 12/2/1956

Rx      Warfarin      5 mg              #60
            1 tab po bid

Ref x 3                              Dr. Andrew Sheen
```

Prescription label:

```
                    Your Friendly Pharmacy
                       1234 Park Avenue
                      Arlington, VA 22209
                 703-243-0036; Fax 703-243-0037
Rx 1002
Brian Waters                        Dr. Shedlock
DOB: 12/2/1956

4433 Simon Blvd, Apt 321, St. Louis, MO 63144
Warfarin      5 mg                  #60
Take one tablet by mouth two times a day.
Refills: 3
```

Identify the error on the prescription label and indicate how it should be corrected.

_____

_____

_____

3. Rx 3:

```
                    Dr. Andrew A. Sheen
                1100 Brentwood Blvd, Suite M780
                    St. Louis, MO 63144
                       314-527-0000
                      DEA FS1234563

Brian Waters                                    January 12, 201X
4433 Simon Blvd, Apt 321, St. Louis, MO 63144
DOB: 12/2/1956

Rx      Lipitor       10 mg             #30
            1 tab po with evening meal

Ref x 5                              Dr. Andrew Sheen
```

Prescription label:

```
                    Your Friendly Pharmacy
                       1234 Park Avenue
                      Arlington, VA 22209
                 703-243-0036; Fax 703-243-0037
Rx 1003                             Date 1/13/201X
Brian Waters                        Dr.Shedlock
DOB: 12/2/1956

4433 Simon Blvd, Apt 321, St. Louis, MO 63144
Lipitor   10 mg                     #30
Take one tablet by mouth with evening meal
Refills: 5
```

Identify the error on the prescription label and indicate how it should be corrected.

_____

_____

_____

4. Rx 4:

```
                    Dr. Andrew A. Sheen
                 1100 Brentwood Blvd, Suite M780
                     St. Louis, MO 63144
                        314-527-0000
                       DEA FS1234563

Brian Waters                              January 12, 201X
4433 Simon Blvd, Apt 321, St. Louis, MO 63144
DOB: 12/2/1956

Rx      Furosemide     40 mg              #30
           1 tab po q am

Ref x 11                              Dr. Andrew Sheen
```

Prescription label:

```
                    Your Friendly Pharmacy
                       1234 Park Avenue
                       Arlington, VA 22209
                  703-243-0036; Fax 703-243-0037

Rx 1004                           Date 1/13/201X
Brian Waters                        Dr. Shedlock
DOB: 12/2/1956

4433 Simon Blvd, Apt 321, St. Louis, MO 63144
Furosemide 40 mg                    #30
Take one tablet by mouth every morning.
Refills: 10
```

Identify the error on the prescription label and indicate how it should be corrected.

_____

_____

_____

5. Rx 5:

```
                    Dr. Andrew A. Sheen
                 1100 Brentwood Blvd, Suite M780
                     St. Louis, MO 63144
                        314-527-0000
                       DEA FS1234563

Brian Waters                              January 12, 201X
4433 Simon Blvd, Apt 321, St. Louis, MO 63144
DOB: 12/2/56

Rx      Cephalexin      500 mg            #30
           1 cap po tid

Ref x 1                              Dr. Andrew Sheen
```

Prescription label:

```
                    Your Friendly Pharmacy
                       1234 Park Avenue
                       Arlington, VA 22209
                  703-243-0036; Fax 703-243-0037

Rx 1005                           Date 1/13/201X
Brian Waters                        Dr. Shedlock
DOB: 10/18/1990

4433 Simon Blvd, Apt 321, St. Louis, MO 63144
Cephalexin      500 mg              #30
Take one capsule by mouth three times a day.
Refills: 1
```

Identify the error on the prescription label and indicate how it should be corrected.

_____

_____

_____

6. Rx 6:

> Dr. Andrew A. Sheen
> 1100 Brentwood Blvd, Suite M780
> St. Louis, MO 63144
> 314-527-0000
> DEA FS1234563
>
> Brian Waters   January 12, 201X
> 4433 Simon Blvd, Apt 321, St. Louis, MO 63144
> DOB: 12/2/1956
>
> Rx   Albuterol Inhaler   17 g   #1
>   1 spray to each nost q 4-6 hr prn asthma
>
> Ref x 11   Dr. Andrew Sheen

Prescription label:

> Your Friendly Pharmacy
> 1234 Park Avenue
> Arlington, VA 22209
> 703-243-0036; Fax 703-243-0037
>
> Rx 1006   Date 1/13/201X
> Brian Waters   Dr. Shedlock
> DOB: 12/2/1956
>
> 4433 Simon Blvd, Apt 321, St. Louis, MO 63144
> Albuterol Inhaler 17 g   #1
> One spray to one nostril every 6-8 hours as needed for asthma.
> Refills: 11

Identify the error on the prescription label and indicate how it should be corrected.

_____

_____

_____

7. Rx 7:

> Dr. Andrew A. Sheen
> 1100 Brentwood Blvd, Suite M780
> St. Louis, MO 63144
> 314-527-0000
> DEA FS1234563
>
> Brian Waters   January 12, 201X
> 4433 Simon Blvd, Apt 321, St. Louis, MO 63144
> DOB: 12/2/1956
>
> Rx   Anucort HC Supp   #12
>   1 supp pr q 12 hr
>
> Ref x 1   Dr. Andrew Sheen

Prescription label:

> Your Friendly Pharmacy
> 1234 Park Avenue
> Arlington, VA 22209
> 703-243-0036; Fax 703-243-0037
>
> Rx 1007   Date 1/13/201X
> Brian Waters   Dr. Shedlock
> DOB: 12/2/1956
>
> 4433 Simon Blvd, Apt 321, St. Louis, MO 63144
> Anucort HC Supp   #12
> Take one suppository by mouth every 12 hours.
> Refills: 1

Identify the error on the prescription label and indicate how it should be corrected.

_____

_____

_____

8. Rx 8:

```
                    Dr. Andrew A. Sheen
                 1100 Brentwood Blvd, Suite M780
                      St. Louis, MO 63144
                         314-527-0000
                        DEA FS1234563

Brian Waters                                    January 12, 201X
4433 Simon Blvd, Apt 321, St. Louis, MO 63144
DOB: 12/2/1956

Rx      Levothyroxine        0.1 mg        #30
         1 tab po q am

Ref x 5                              Dr. Andrew Sheen
```

Prescription label:

```
                    Your Friendly Pharmacy
                      1234 Park Avenue
                      Arlington, VA 22209
                  703-243-0036; Fax 703-243-0037

Rx 1008                          Date 1/13/201X
Brian Waters                        Dr. Shedlock
DOB:  12/2/1956

4433 Simon Blvd, Apt 321, St. Louis, MO 63144
Levothyroxine    0.1 mg                #30
1 tab po q am.

Refills: 5
```

Identify the error on the prescription label and indicate how it should be corrected.

_____

_____

_____

9. Rx 9:

```
                    Dr. Andrew A. Sheen
                 1100 Brentwood Blvd, Suite M780
                      St. Louis, MO 63144
                         314-527-0000
                        DEA FS1234563

Brian Waters                                    January 12, 201X
4433 Simon Blvd, Apt 321, St. Louis, MO 63144
DOB: 12/2/1956

Rx      Nitrostat      1/150 gr      #25
         1 tab sl prn angina attack, may repeat every 5 minutes upto 5 times per attack

Ref x prn                            Dr. Andrew Sheen
```

Prescription label:

```
                    Your Friendly Pharmacy
                      1234 Park Avenue
                      Arlington, VA 22209
                  703-243-0036; Fax 703-243-0037

Rx 1009                          12/13/201X
Brian Waters                        Dr. Shedlock
DOB: 12/2/1956

4433 Simon Blvd, Apt 321, St. Louis, MO 63144
Nitrostat        1/150              #25
Take one tablet by mouth as needed for angina attack; may repeat every 5 minutes upto 5 times per attack.

Refills: prn
```

Identify the error on the prescription label and indicate how it should be corrected.

_____

_____

_____

10. Rx 10:

```
                    Dr. Andrew A. Sheen
                1100 Brentwood Blvd, Suite M780
                    St. Louis, MO 63144
                       314-527-0000
                      DEA FS1234563

Brian Waters                              January 12, 201X
4433 Simon Blvd, Apt 321, St. Louis, MO 63144
DOB: 12/2/1956

Rx     Alprazolam 1 mg                #90
       1 tab po q 8 hr prn anxiety

Ref x 2                          Dr. Andrew Sheen
```

Prescription label:

```
                  Your Friendly Pharmacy
                     1234 Park Avenue
                    Arlington, VA 22209
               703-243-0036; Fax 703-243-0037

Rx 1010                         Date 1/13/201X
Brian Waters
DOB: 12/2/1956

4433 Simon Blvd, Apt 321, St. Louis, MO 63144
Alprazolam      1 mg            #90
Take one tablet by mouth three times a day as needed for anxiety.

Refills: 2
```

Identify the error on the prescription label and indicate how it should be corrected.

_____

_____

_____

Customer Service

Objective: To emphasize the importance of customer service in the practice of pharmacy.

> The pharmacist and the pharmacy technician assist patients in their treatment through the use of medication and information. During their interaction with the patient, it is vital that they listen carefully to the patient. They must be able to explain things to the patient in words the patient can understand. In addition to the words that are used, the pharmacist and the pharmacy technician must be aware of their body language and what it conveys to the patient. Empathy should be conveyed to the patient.
>
> Customer service issues occur every day. Many of these issues could have been avoided if the customer had been acknowledged in a timely manner and treated properly. Common complaints by the patient include the wait time for a prescription to be processed, being out of stock of a medication, and issues caused through billing of their prescription to their third-party prescription carrier. A pharmacy technician must be able to assist in finding solutions to problems that arise in the practice of pharmacy.

Lab Activity #7.5: Read each of the following scenarios. Explain how you would resolve the issue and why you made that decision.

Equipment needed:

- Paper
- Pencil/pen

Time needed to complete this activity: 45 minutes

1. Kathy Kraisinger brings her empty prescription bottle of hydrochlorothiazide 5 mg into the pharmacy for a refill on Saturday afternoon at 4 PM. No refills are indicated on the bottle. You call the physician's office for a refill, but the office has closed for the day and will not reopen until Monday morning at 8 AM. What will you do and why?

_____

_____

_____

_____

_____

2. You are entering a patient's prescription into your computer system and have submitted the prescription to the patient's prescription provider. The prescription is rejected by the prescription provider with the following explanation "INVALID ID NUMBER/INVALID GROUP NUMBER." How would you handle the situation?

_____

_____

_____

_____

_____

3. Bill Kunze is picking up his prescription at Preston's Pharmacy. The pharmacy technician notices that a prescription for Bill's wife has been filled and is in the prescription bins. What will you do and why?

_____

_____

_____

_____

_____

4. Tom Dagit brings in a prescription for Dilaudid 2 mg #30. The pharmacy technician checks for the amount of Dilaudid 2 mg on hand and notices that the pharmacy is temporarily out of stock. What will you do and why?

_____

_____

_____

_____

_____

5. You are processing a prescription for a patient, and the prescription is rejected by the prescription provider with the following explanation "REFILL TOO SOON." You inform the patient of the situation, and he tells you he is leaving on vacation tomorrow for 3 weeks. How would you handle this situation?

_____

_____

_____

_____

_____

6. A patient comes to the pharmacy counter and asks you where she can find a bottle of ibuprofen to purchase. What will you do and why?

_____

_____

_____

_____

_____

7. What will you say when you are answering the pharmacy's telephone?

_____

_____

_____

_____

_____

8. A patient comes to the pharmacy and asks you to recommend an allergy medication. What would you do and why?

_____

_____

_____

_____

_____

9. You are the only technician working with the pharmacist today. The pharmacist has asked you to accept patients' prescriptions at the drug counter. A patient approaches the drug counter at the same time the telephone begins to ring. How will you handle this situation?

_____

_____

_____

_____

10. A Hispanic patient brings in a new prescription to be filled at the pharmacy. When you ask the patient for his address and insurance information, you learn that he does not speak English. Neither the pharmacist nor you are able to speak Spanish. How would you handle this situation?

_____

_____

_____

_____

_____

11. You are filling a prescription for a patient and receive the following rejection message from the prescription provider: "DRUG NOT ON FORMULARY." How would you handle the situation?

_____

_____

_____

_____

_____

12. It is Friday afternoon at 4 PM, and you are ringing up customers' prescriptions at the cash register. A total of 11 people are waiting in line to drop off or pick up their prescriptions. How would you handle the situation? Why?

_____

_____

_____

_____

_____

13. A woman found a prescription for penicillin for her boyfriend from the community's sexually transmitted disease clinic. The prescription was filled at the pharmacy 2 days ago, and she would like to know what it is used to treat. What would you tell her?

_____

_____

_____

_____

_____

14. A mother is dropping off a prescription at the pharmacy with her sixth grade son. As they are waiting for the prescription to be filled, the son asks you what the difference is between prescription and over-the-counter medications. How would you explain this to him?

_____

_____

_____

_____

15. A patient comes to the pharmacy and asks for a box of pseudoephedrine that is kept at the pharmacy. You ask to see his driver's license as a form of identification. The patient becomes extremely upset with your request and states that at other pharmacies they do not have this requirement. How would you handle the situation?

_____

_____

_____

_____

_____

16. A patient appears to be upset as she hands you a prescription for a terminal illness for which she has been diagnosed. Would you demonstrate sympathy or empathy toward the patient? Why?

_____

_____

_____

_____

_____

TERMS AND DEFINITIONS

Select the correct term from the following list and write the corresponding letter in the blank next to the statement.

A. Analgesic
B. Antiinflammatory
C. Antiseptic
D. Antitussive
E. Acetylsalicylic acid
F. Bulk forming
G. Expectorant
H. Prophylaxis
I. ROA
J. Sunscreen

_____ 1. A substance that stops or slows the growth of microorganisms on surfaces such as skin

_____ 2. Route of administration

_____ 3. Medication that causes loss of sensation/pain due to interruption in the nervous system pathway between the organ and the brain

_____ 4. Aspirin

_____ 5. A drug that thins respiratory secretions, allowing the patient to cough up mucus from the lungs

_____ 6. A substance that protects the skin from ultraviolet (UV) light, thus protecting from sunburn; the skin protection factor (SPF) rates effectiveness

_____ 7. A drug that reduces swelling, redness, and pain and promotes healing

_____ 8. Fiber used to add bulk to the stool to relieve constipation or used to cause a feeling of fullness to reduce appetite

_____ 9. Treatment given before a possible event to prevent the event from happening

_____ 10. A drug that can reduce the coughing reflex

TRUE OR FALSE

Write T or F next to each statement.

_____ 1. The ability to buy drugs over-the-counter can lead to substantial savings for customers.

_____ 2. Most OTC drug labels recommend dosages for children younger than 2 years.

_____ 3. Adverse reaction reports are required for both prescription and OTC drugs.

_____ 4. Very few agents are 100% pure.

_____ 5. The *potency* of a medication refers to the ability of the drug to produce a given effect.

_____ 6. *Bioavailability* is the amount of drug made available to the bloodstream or target tissue once absorbed into the body.

_____ 7. *Efficacy* is the ability of a drug to produce the desired effect in the body.

_____ 8. Standards of safety and effectiveness are lower for OTC drugs than for legend drugs.

_____ 9. Sunburn and acne are very serious skin conditions and should not be treated at home.

_____ 10. Strep throat can be treated with OTC medications.

MULTIPLE CHOICE

Complete each question by circling the best answer.

1. The number of OTC drugs available to consumers has increased since the:
   A. 1960s
   B. 1970s
   C. 1980s
   D. 1990s

2. Drug companies know that consumers want more OTC drugs available to them so that they can:
   A. Save money
   B. Be involved in their own treatment
   C. Both A and B
   D. None of the above

3. Which of the following is *not* a category applied by the FDA to rate OTC drugs before they are allowed to enter the market?
   A. Safe and effective for the claimed therapeutic indication
   B. Not recognized as safe and effective
   C. Additional data need to be obtained to determine safety and efficacy
   D. Toxic; no additional data needed

4. The FDA regulates aspects affecting the safety of OTC medications; the aspects regulated are:
   A. Purity and potency
   B. Bioavailability and efficacy
   C. Safety and toxicity
   D. All of the above

5. New OTC drugs must go through certain phases before approval. The phase during which a final review is done on the ingredients of a drug and the public is allowed to give feedback is known as:
   A. Phase 1
   B. Phase 2
   C. Phase 3
   D. Phase 4

6. A *monograph* includes:
   A. Information about a drug
   B. Descriptive information about clinical trials
   C. The structure of the chemical compound
   D. All of the above

7. Which condition cannot be treated with OTC drugs?
   A. High blood pressure
   B. Fever
   C. Cough
   D. Diarrhea

8. Children and teenagers should not take aspirin for chickenpox or flu, because it has been associated with:
   A. Toxic shock syndrome
   B. Reye's syndrome
   C. Sudden infant death syndrome
   D. Acquired immunodeficiency syndrome

9. *NSAID* stands for:
   A. Nonsafety caps for AIDS patients
   B. Not safe as an IUD service
   C. Nonsteroidal antiinflammatory drug
   D. Nonsteroidal antiinflammatory disease

10. A common side effect of first-generation antihistamines is:
    A. Drowsiness
    B. Diarrhea
    C. Agitation
    D. Constipation

SHORT ANSWER

Write a short response to each question in the space provided.

1. Give three examples of antiinflammatory products.

   A. _____

   B. _____

   C. _____

2. Which decongestant does not cause drowsiness? _____

3. What is the most common nonprescription agent used in hospitals to help patients sleep? _____

4. Give two classes of drugs used to reduce or relieve gastric acid secretions.

   A. _____

   B. _____

5. Into which layer of skin does a diabetic person inject insulin? _____

6. How do sunscreens and sun blocks work?

   A. Sunscreens

   _____

   _____

   B. Sun blocks

   _____

   _____

7. What is the most common OTC product recommended to help dry out pimples? _____

8. Basic skin care for acne involves _____

_____.

9. Approximately how many OTC products are on the market today? _____

MATCHING

Match the term in the left column with the alternative name in the right column.

_____ 1. Urticaria

_____ 2. Genital warts

_____ 3. Tinea pedis

_____ 4. Canker sores

_____ 5. Cold sores

A. Herpes simplex virus
B. Small topical ulcers
C. Hives
D. Human papillomavirus
E. Athlete's foot

RESEARCH ACTIVITY

Follow the instructions given in each exercise and provide a response.

1. Access the website *www.fda.gov*. In the Quick Info Links section, locate Drugs@FDA; type in OTC. Investigate what legend drugs have been converted to OTC status.

2. Access the website *www.accutanehelp.com*.

   A. What are some of the serious side effects of the acne product Accutane?

   B. What precautions should be taken by patients using this skin care product?

CRITICAL THINKING

Reply to each question based on what you have learned in the chapter.

1. In a chain store or mass merchandiser outlet, where is the pharmacy located? Why?

2. You have a sore throat, and none of the OTC lozenges are helping. You have been told to gargle with saltwater. How will this help your sore throat?

3. Sometimes people buy an OTC medication because someone they know tried it and it worked for that person. Why should you not base your decision to buy OTC medications on that reasoning?

4. The FDA recently allowed Prilosec to become an OTC product. What other drugs do you think should become OTC medications, provided they are safe and effective for patients?

5. Tanning beds, air-brushed tans, and tans in a bottle are very popular products. What are the dangers of overusing some of these products on your skin? What advice would you give people you know who are overusing these products?

LAB SCENARIOS

Over-the-Counter (OTC) Medications

Objective: To introduce the pharmacy technician to various over-the-counter medications and their indication(s), warning(s), dosage form(s), and route(s) of administration.

Lab Activity #8.1: Visit a local pharmacy and familiarize yourself with the OTC section of the store. Complete the following table of OTC products.

Equipment needed:

- Retail pharmacy
- Pencil/pen

Time needed to complete the exercise: 60 minutes

Brand (Trade) Name	Active Ingredient(s)	Medication Strength	Indication	Warning(s)	Dosage Form(s) Available	Route(s) of Administration
A-200						
Abreva						
Advil						
Afrin						
Alavert						
Aleve						
Ambesol						
Bayer Aspirin						
BC Headache Powder						
Benadryl						
Benefiber						
Betadine						
Bufferin						
Caltrate 600						
Citrucel Powder						
Claritin Reditabs						
Claritin-D						
Clearazil						

Brand (Trade) Name	Active Ingredient(s)	Medication Strength	Indication	Warning(s)	Dosage Form(s) Available	Route(s) of Administration
Contac						
Debrox Drops						
Delsym Extended-Release 12-Hour Cough Suppressant						
Dimetapp						
Dimetapp-DM						
Domeboro						
Dulcolax						
Ecotrin						
Excedrin Extra Strength						
Ex-Lax						
Feosol						
FiberCon						
Gas-X						
Gaviscon						
Gly-Oxide						
Gyne-Lotrimin						
Imodium A-D						
Lactaid						
Lamisil						
Lotrimin						
Maalox						
Metamucil						
Mineral Ice						
Monistat 7						
Motrin IB						

Continued

Brand (Trade) Name	Active Ingredient(s)	Medication Strength	Indication	Warning(s)	Dosage Form(s) Available	Route(s) of Administration
Mylanta						
Neosporin						
NicoDerm						
Nicorette						
Nizoral A-D						
Nytol						
OsCal						
Pepcid A-C						
Pepto-Bismol						
Phazyme						
Polysporin						
Preparation H						
Prilosec						
Robitussin						
Rogaine						
Sudafed						
Tagamet HB						
TheraFlu						
Tinactin						
Triaminic						
Tums						
Tylenol						
Vicks 44D						
Vicks Dayquil						
Vicks Nyquil						

TERMS AND DEFINITIONS

Select the correct term from the following list and write the corresponding letter in the blank next to the statement.

A. Antiemetic
B. Antihypertensive
C. Ayurveda
D. Chiropractic
E. Diagnosis
F. Fat-soluble
G. Herb
H. Homeopathy
I. Placebo
J. Synthetic
K. Tincture

_____ 1. An inert compound thought to be an active agent

_____ 2. A holistic medical system that originated in India

_____ 3. A system of therapy based on the belief that medicinal substances that cause a specific symptom can be used to treat an illness that yields the same symptoms

_____ 4. A physician's assessment of the cause of a condition

_____ 5. Drugs that are absorbed into the body's fat layer

_____ 6. Plant extract mixed with alcohol

_____ 7. Manual manipulation of the joints and muscles

_____ 8. Agents that stop nausea and vomiting

_____ 9. Medication made in a laboratory

_____ 10. Agent that reduces blood pressure

_____ 11. Any herbaceous plant consisting of fleshy stems

TRUE OR FALSE

Write T or F next to each statement.

_____ 1. Traditional medicine has been in existence for thousands of years, whereas alternative approaches have been practiced for only a few hundred years.

_____ 2. Western medicine relies on scientific methods to prove the effectiveness of treatments.

_____ 3. Developing countries use herbs as their main form of treatment.

_____ 4. Herbs are considered a form of traditional medication.

_____ 5. Self-hypnosis was found clinically to reduce the pain of surgery in patients.

_____ 6. A placebo contains no active ingredients.

_____ 7. Biofeedback should be practiced only with a biofeedback instructor present.

_____ 8. Chiropractic therapy usually requires many treatment sessions.

_____ 9. Crystal healing is a well-documented, scientific study of overcoming illnesses.

_____ 10. Herbs are natural and therefore are not harmful.

_____ 11. Herbs that are brewed for teas usually are more potent than those prepared in capsule form.

_____ 12. Many physicians and scientists consider spiritual healing a testimonial to the power of the placebo effect.

Complete the question by circling the best answer.

1. Traditional medicine includes all of the following except:
   A. Physician visits
   B. Prescription drugs
   C. Laboratory tests
   D. Visits to a chiropractor

2. Complementary alternative medicine includes all of the following except:
   A. Herbs
   B. X-rays
   C. Acupuncture
   D. Yoga

3. Controversial therapies include:
   A. Crystal healing
   B. Spiritual healing
   C. Magnetic healing
   D. All of the above

4. Eastern medicine includes treatments originating from all of the following *except:*
   A. Eastern Asia
   B. India
   C. Eastern United States
   D. Far East countries

5. The beginning of the golden age of microbiology is considered to be the:
   A. 1600s
   B. 1700s
   C. 1800s
   D. 1900s

6. A reason people may turn to alternative medicines is:
   A. Risk of drug side effects
   B. Rising cost of drugs
   C. Diseases for which no medications are available
   D. All of the above

7. Which of the following is *not* considered a nondrug treatment?
   A. Massage
   B. Herbs
   C. Meditation
   D. Biofeedback

8. Herbs used in Chinese medicine can:
   A. Cure the body of illness
   B. Prevent future problems
   C. A and B
   D. None of the above

9. Biofeedback has proved effective for all of the following *except:*
   A. Love life
   B. Heart rate
   C. Hypertension
   D. Gastrointestinal activity

10. Chiropractic treatment can include all of the following *except:*
    A. Adjustments of the joints
    B. Chemotherapy
    C. Massage
    D. Heat therapy

11. To treat a minor burn, a patient could use:
    A. Aloe vera
    B. Chamomile
    C. Garlic
    D. Ginkgo biloba

12. The belief that if a small amount of the substance that caused a person's disease or condition is consumed, it will enable the body to fight off the disease, is known as:
    A. The placebo effect
    B. Ayurveda
    C. Homeopathy
    D. Spiritual healing

FILL IN THE BLANK

Answer each question by completing the statement in the space provided.

1. From which plant is the heart drug digoxin made? _____

2. What form of alternative medicine uses needles inserted at specific points throughout the body? _____

3. The heart of Chinese medicine is the _____ and _____, which represent both _____ and _____ entities.

4. Art therapy is used extensively in _____ with _____.

5. Ayurveda is based on a person's knowing his or her _____ _____.

6. Chiropractic therapy is an _____ approach to treating pain from _____ _____ ____ _____ of bones.

7. The FDA does not regulate herbs as drugs because they are considered to be a _____ _____.

Chapter **9** Complementary and Alternative Medicine

MATCHING

Match the following herbs with their treatment targets.

_____ 1. Black cohosh

_____ 2. Chamomile

_____ 3. Ginger

_____ 4. Milk thistle

_____ 5. Echinacea

_____ 6. Garlic

_____ 7. Ginkgo biloba

_____ 8. Ginseng

_____ 9. St. John's wort

_____ 10. Valerian

A. Promote sleep
B. Overall wellness
C. Colds and infections
D. Mood
E. Flatulence, gastrointestinal disturbances
F. Support circulation, memory
G. Nausea, vertigo
H. Liver health
I. Support hormonal changes
J. Support heart health

SHORT ANSWER

Write a short response to each question in the space provided.

1. The holistic approach to diagnosis and treatments includes _____, _____, and even _____.

2. What are the three main goals of NCCAM?

   A. _____

   B. _____

   C. _____

3. Complementary medicine is the use of _____ therapies and _____ medicine together.

4. Who oversees the manufacture of homeopathic drugs? _____

5. Homeopathic drugs are in the same category as _____ drugs.

6. Why is it important to know the family name of an herb? _____

   _____

7. What is the premise of homeopathy? _____

   _____

RESEARCH ACTIVITY

Follow the instructions given in each exercise and provide a response.

1. Access the website *www.rxlist.com*. Locate the list, Top 30 Western Herbs. Print the list and compare the various herbs and treatments with those discussed in the chapter.

2. Access the website *www.altmedicine.com*. What is the purpose of this website?

3. Access the website *http://nccam.nih.gov/health*. Read the information given under Understanding Complementary and Alternative Medicine (CAM).

REFLECT CRITICALLY

CRITICAL THINKING

Reply to each question based on what you have learned in the chapter.

1. Alternative medicine has been on the rise the past few years. Many people are not aware that the FDA does not regulate many of the "natural" products being marketed. As a consumer, how can you be sure that these "natural" products really contain the ingredients reported on the labels?

2. Besides the various therapies and herbal products discussed in the chapter, what other forms of alternative medicine are available?

3. Spiritual healing brings another dimension to alternative medicine. Why is it so different from the other forms discussed in the chapter?

4. You are trying to convince your classmates that trying alternative medicine is better than seeing a physician every time you feel ill. How would you make your case for this form of therapy?

LAB SCENARIOS

Complementary Alternative Medicine

Objective: To introduce the pharmacy technician to complementary alternative medicine and its usage in the prevention and treatment of illness.

> Complementary and alternative medication is defined as a "group of diverse medical and health care systems, practices and products that are not generally considered part of conventional medicine." Conventional medicine is medicine practiced by holders of M.D. and O.D. degrees and by all allied health professionals. Complementary and alternative medicine is gaining in popularity in the United States. As a member of the allied health team, pharmacy technicians need to be familiar with complementary and alternative medicine because of the changing demographics of our society.

Lab Activity #9.1: Using the National Center for Complementary and Alternative Medicine website *(www.nccam .nih.gov)*, complete the following table of herbal products.

Equipment needed:

- Computer with Internet access
- Pencil/pen
- Paper

Time needed to complete this activity: 45 minutes

Herbal Product	Common Names	Latin Name	Indication	FDA-Approved Use	List Two Side Effects	List One Contraindication
Aloe Vera						
Astragalus						
Bilberry						
Bitter Orange						
Black Cohosh						
Cat's Claw						
Chamomile						
Chasteberry						
Cranberry						
Dandelion						

Herbal Product	Common Names	Latin Name	Indication	FDA-Approved Use	List Two Side Effects	List One Contraindication
Echinacea						
Ephedra						
European Elder						
Evening Primrose Oil						
Fenugeek						
Feverfew						
Flaxseed						
Garlic						
Ginger						
Ginkgo						
Ginseng						
Hawthorn						
Hoodia						
Horse Chestnut						
Kava						
Lavender						
Licorice Root						
Milk Thistle						
Mistletoe						

Continued

Chapter **9** **Complementary and Alternative Medicine**

Herbal Product	Common Names	Latin Name	Indication	FDA-Approved Use	List Two Side Effects	List One Contraindication
Noni						
Peppermint Oil						
Red Clover						
Saw Palmetto						
Soy						
St. John's Wort						
Thunder God Vine						
Tumeric						
Valerian						
Yohimbe						

Lab Activity #9.2: Using the National Center for Complementary and Alternative Medicine website *(www.nccam.nih. gov),* answer the following questions on complementary and alternative treatments.

Equipment needed:

- Computer with Internet access
- Pencil/pen
- Paper

Time needed to complete this activity: 60 minutes

1. Acupuncture

   a. Where did acupuncture originate?

   _____

   b. What two opposing and inseparable forces are being balanced?

   _____

   c. What does Yin represent?

   _____

   d. What does Yang represent?

   _____

e. Approximately how many people in the United States receive acupuncture each year?

_____

f. Who regulates the needles used in acupuncture?

_____

g. Does an acupuncture practitioner require a license to practice in the United States?

_____

h. Would you consider acupuncture as a therapy? Why or why not?

_____

_____

_____

2. Aromatherapy

   a. What are two examples of essential oils that may be used in aromatherapy?

_____

_____

   b. What is one theory of how aromatherapy works in the treatment of symptoms and side effects of cancer therapy?

_____

_____

_____

   c. What are two routes of administration for essential oils?

_____

   d. What is one side effect that may be experienced by an individual undergoing aromatherapy?

_____

   e. Would you consider aromatherapy as a therapy? Why or why not?

_____

_____

_____

3. Ayurvedic Medicine

   a. Where did Ayurvedic medication originate?

_____

   b. What is the goal of Ayurvedic medicine?

_____

_____

   c. What does the term *Ayurveda* mean?

_____

d. What are the eight branches of Ayurvedic medicine?

_____

_____

e. How many Americans use Ayurvedic medicine each year?

_____

f. What two concepts does Ayurvedic medicine involve?

_____

_____

g. What is a *dosha*?

_____

_____

h. What do the three dosha represent?

_____

_____

_____

i. What are four treatment practices used in Ayurvedic medicine?

_____

_____

j. What are two concerns regarding Ayurvedic medications?

_____

_____

k. Would you use Ayurvedic medicine? Why or why not?

_____

_____

_____

4. Chiropractic

a. On what area of the body does chiropractic practice focus?

_____

_____

b. What does the term *chiropractic* mean?

_____

c. What percentage of American adults have used chiropractic alignments within the past year?

_____

d. What requirements must an individual possess to practice as a chiropractor?

_____

_____

_____

e. Who regulates the chiropractic practice?

_____

_____

f. Would you use a chiropractor to treat a condition? Why or why not?

_____

_____

_____

5. Massage

a. What is massage therapy?

_____

_____

b. How many Americans receive a massage each year?

_____

c. What conditions may be treated by using massage therapy?

_____

_____

d. What are five licenses or certifications that a massage therapist may possess?

_____

_____

_____

_____

e. Would you use massage therapy to treat a condition? Why or why not?

_____

_____

_____

6. Meditation

a. Why might a patient use meditation as a form of treatment?

_____

_____

Chapter **9** **Complementary and Alternative Medicine**

b. What are the four elements of meditations?

_____

_____

_____

_____

c. How many Americans have meditated within the past year?

_____

d. Where does Mindfulness originate?

_____

e. Where does Transcendental Meditation originate?

_____

f. What is hypothesized as the mechanism of action for meditation?

_____

_____

_____

g. Do you meditate? If yes, how has it helped you?

_____

_____

_____

7. Naturopathy

a. Where did naturopathy originate?

_____

b. How many Americans participate in naturopathy?

_____

c. What are the six principles of naturopathy?

_____

_____

_____

_____

d. What type of education does a naturopathic physician require?

_____

e. How many states have licensing requirements for naturopathic physicians?

_____

f. What methods of treatment does a naturopathic physician use?

_____

_____

_____

g. Would you use a naturopathic physician? Why or why not?

_____

_____

_____

_____

8. Reiki

a. Where did Reiki originate?

_____

b. What does the term *Reiki* mean?

_____

c. What is the belief behind Reiki?

_____

_____

d. How many Americans use Reiki?

_____

e. Is training required for Reiki?

_____

f. Would you use Reiki? Why or why not?

_____

_____

_____

_____

9. Tai Chi

a. Where did Tai Chi originate?

_____

b. What does Tai Chi mean?

_____

c. What Chinese concepts does Tai Chi use?

_____

_____

d. How many Americans use Tai Chi?

_____

135

e. Why do individuals practice Tai Chi?

_____

_____

_____

_____

f. Would you use Tai Chi as a form of treatment? Why or why not?

_____

_____

_____

_____

10. Yoga

a. Where did yoga originate?

_____

b. What techniques are used in yoga?

_____

_____

c. What percentage of adults in the United States practice yoga?

_____

d. What is Iyengar yoga?

_____

_____

e. What is Ashtanga yoga?

_____

_____

f. What is Vini yoga?

_____

_____

g. What is Kundalini yoga?

_____

_____

h. What is Bikram yoga?

_____

_____

i. Would you use yoga as a form of therapy? Why or why not?

_____

_____

_____

_____

TERMS AND DEFINITIONS

Select the correct term from the following list and write the corresponding letter in the blank next to the statement.

A. Aseptic technique
B. Crash cart
C. PAR
D. Investigational drug
E. NKDA
F. Satellite pharmacy
G. Sure-Med
H. prn
I. Protocol
J. Stat order

_____E_____ 1. No known drug allergy

_____I_____ 2. Set of standards and guidelines by which the facility works

_____G_____ 3. Automated dispensing system often used in hospitals

_____H_____ 4. As needed

_____D_____ 5. Drug not approved yet by the FDA for marketing, but is in clinical trials

_____F_____ 6. Smaller pharmacy located in hospital away from the central pharmacy

_____C_____ 7. Periodic Automatic Replenishment

_____A_____ 8. Method of preventing contamination by organisms

_____J_____ 9. Must be filled as soon as possible, usually within 5 to 15 minutes

_____B____10. Contains trays of medications, administration sets, oxygen, and other materials used for life-threatening situations

TRUE OR FALSE

Write T or F next to each statement.

___T___ 1. A hospital pharmacy is one of the most challenging areas in which a pharmacy technician can work.

___F___ 2. Hospital pharmacies have more job openings than community pharmacies.

___T___ 3. Large hospitals may have a central pharmacy and smaller satellite pharmacies throughout the hospital.

___T___ 4. Satellite pharmacies stock specific medications for the ward they service to speed up the turnaround time on medication orders.

___F___ 5. All hospitals must meet only state guidelines.

___T___ 6. The board of pharmacy has the authority to impose fines and to close down pharmacies.

___T___ 7. Technicians must have scheduling flexibility because they will need to work all shifts, including weekends and holidays.

___F___ 8. All medications are delivered to the patient floors using one cart that is rotated daily.

___T___ 9. A hospital pharmacy must stock a wide variety of medications in many dosage forms.

___F___10. When nurses call the pharmacy, the most common question is, "Where are the meds I ordered?"

___F___11. Automated systems used in hospitals are replacing technicians.

___T___12. A hospital pharmacy technician should be an energetic, multitasking-type person.

___F___13. When unit dose medications are prepared, the final check is done by the lead technician.

___T___14. The Joint Commission now requires hospitals to make all medications patient-dose specific.

___T___15. The task of counting and tracking controlled substances is a critical job that requires perfection.

Complete each question by circling the best answer.

1. The policies and procedures handbook contains information about:
   A. Mandatory training
   B. Cafeteria menus
   C. Physicians' orders
   D. All of the above

2. Factors that differentiate hospitals include:
   A. Outpatient services
   B. Diagnostic capabilities
   C. Surgical procedures
   D. All of the above

3. One of the agencies that govern the operation of hospitals is the:
   A. HFC
   B. HCFA
   C. RPH
   D. ICU

4. All necessary information included on a patient's admitting record to ensure that orders are filled correctly is provided by:
   A. A physician or nurse
   B. A unit clerk
   C. Both A and B
   D. Pharmacy staff

5. When patients with the same last name end up on the same floor, which auxiliary label should be used?
   A. Take as directed
   B. Name alert
   C. May cause drowsiness
   D. Shake well

6. IV medication order labels show the:
   A. Drug name, strength, and dosage form
   B. Route of administration and scheduled dosing time
   C. Patient's name, medical record number, and room number
   D. All of the above

7. The technician responsible for filling med drawers for patients currently in the hospital is a(n):
   A. IV technician
   B. Satellite technician
   C. Unit dose cart fill technician
   D. Floor stock technician

8. In a horizontal flow hood, the airflow pattern is in what direction?
    A. From the back of the hood to the front
    B. From the top of the hood to the bottom
    C. From the bottom of the hood to the top
    D. From the front of the hood to the back

9. The inventory control technician is not responsible for:
    A. Ordering stock
    B. Checking off other technicians' work
    C. Billing
    D. Restocking shelves

10. Which of the following is *not* an automated hospital system?
    A. Pyxis
    B. SureMed
    C. Robot RX
    D. TJC

11. Standing orders are:
    A. Prescriptions waiting to be picked up
    B. Orders written by an intern or resident
    C. Written protocols for drugs used in a specific situation
    D. Order given to a pharmacy technician for pharmacist approval

12. Point of entry systems provide electronic access to:
    A. Medical and drug information data
    B. Secure entry into the pharmacy
    C. Pyxis machine
    D. Hospital supply room

13. Using the computerized prescriber order entry, a _____ can enter all labs, dietary requirements, medi-
    cations, and special notes into the computer.
    A. Nurse
    B. Physician
    C. Unit clerk
    D. Pharmacy technician

14. Enforceable regulations for IV preparations have been provided by the:
    A. Joint Commission
    B. Board of Pharmacy
    C. United States Pharmacopeia-797
    D. *Physicians' Desk Reference*

15. Examples of prime vendors for ordering pharmacy supplies include:
    A. McKesson
    B. Cardinal Health
    C. AmerisourceBergen
    D. All of the above

FILL IN THE BLANK

Answer each question by completing the statement in the space provided.

1. _____ technique is extremely important is preparing all IV medications or other sterile products, such as _____, _____, and compounded ophthalmics.

2. When preparing chemotherapy, a technician must wear a _____ and _____ gloves.

3. The proper placement of labels is important to _____ _____ of the _____ _____ and its contents.

4. All controlled substances are counted _____ times daily on the nursing units.

5. The _____ levels are the quantities of medications that should be kept on the nursing unit ("floor") at all times.

6. Only _____ can sign in controlled substances to the nursing unit.

7. _____ is a term used to define the guidelines in a hospital setting, such as the type of medication available for dispensing.

8. Specialty technician tasks include assisting with _____ _____ and _____ therapy.

9. If the hospital uses an automated medication dispensing system, there may be no need for a _____.

10. The three types of stat trays stocked for code carts by hospital pharmacies are _____, _____, and _____.

SHORT ANSWER

Write a short response to each question in the space provided.

1. List three duties of the inventory control technician.

   A. _____

   B. _____

   C. _____

2. What three specialty departments in an institution (hospital) stock many drugs in injectable forms, as well as a variety of oral and injectable controlled substances?

   A. _____

   B. _____

   C. _____

3. Stat orders can be filled in _____ minutes and if possible can be _____ to

ensure that they get to the correct destination _____ and _____.

4. When a technician is working inside a horizontal flow hood, the orientation of the hands _____.

5. For what are the following governmental agencies responsible?

A. TJC _____

B. HCFA _____

C. BOP _____

RESEARCH ACTIVITY

Follow the instructions given in each exercise and provide a response.

1. Access *www.ptcb.org* and look up the duties of a hospital technician.

2. Visit or call a local hospital pharmacy and interview the following hospital technicians: IV therapy, chemotherapy, UD fill, and controlled substance technicians. Ask the following questions:

A. What are your job duties?

B. What training did you receive?

C. What is the most satisfying part of your job?

CRITICAL THINKING

Reply to each question based on what you have learned in the chapter.

1. Many technicians work in inpatient hospital pharmacies because the pay scale is higher than that found in retail or community pharmacies. What are some other reasons a technician might want to work in an inpatient hospital pharmacy?

   Room to advance in career and being cross-trained in other dept's. There are many avenues to move up in pay scale and responsibility.

2. The job descriptions of inpatient pharmacy technicians are changing because of the various automated systems coming into use to fill medication carts. Outline a job description for an automated dispensing technician.

   Fill up/stock all patient orders and dose out the proper medications. Stock crash cart, able to take inventory w/ what drugs someone has and what they need.

3. The relationship between nursing and pharmacy staffs can be tumultuous at times. How can you, as a technician, foster a better relationship between these two groups of professionals?

   Always be courteous and respectful and prioritize hospital tasks accordingly.

LAB SCENARIOS

Hospital Pharmacy

Automated dispensing systems are used in hospital pharmacies and result in improved patient care. Automation speeds up the dispensing process, resulting in fewer medication errors and improved patient outcomes. Computer dispensing systems allow for improved inventory management by the institution, resulting in fewer dollars invested in the pharmacy's inventory. Many of the tasks previously performed in the pharmacy by an individual were time consuming and had a high potential for error. Technology enables the role of both the pharmacist and the pharmacy technician to continue to evolve.

Lab Activity #10.1: Order up-to quantity

Equipment needed:

- Calculator
- Pencil/pen

Time needed to complete this activity: 10 minutes

1. Calculate the number of full bottles of medication you would order to meet the order up-to quantity of each medication.

Medication	Package Size	Quantity on Hand (Bottles)	Desired Quantity (Bottles)	Number of Bottles Ordered
Albuterol Inhaler (200 sprays)	1	45	75	
Alprazolam 0.5 mg	1000	1	2.5	
Amitriptyline 50 mg	500	1.75	2	
Amlodipine 10 mg	500	3	2	
Amoxicillin 500 mg	500	2.5	4.25	
Cephalexin 500 mg	500	3.25	3.75	
Furosemide 40 mg	1000	2.75	4	
Hydrochlorothiazide 50 mg	1000	0.75	3.5	
Hydrocodone 5 mg/ Acetaminophen 500 mg	500	1	2	
Levothyroxine 0.1 mg	1000	2.75	3.25	
Lexapro 10 mg	90	3.05	4.25	
Lisinopril 10 mg	1000	0.95	1.8	
Metoprolol 50 mg	1000	0.25	2.75	
Potassium Chloride 8 mEq	500	2	3.5	
Propranolol 40 mg	1000	3	5.5	
Serevent Inhaler (120 sprays)	1	34	52	
Simvastatin 40 mg	1000	1.75	2.8	
Singulair 10 mg	8000	0.75	1.25	
Warfarin 5 mg	1000	3.25	4.5	
Zolpidem 5 mg	500	0.75	1.25	

Lab Activity #10.2: Perpetual inventory of controlled substances

Equipment needed:

- Calculator
- Pencil/pen
- Paper

Time needed to complete this activity: 10 minutes

The hospital pharmacy has received the following orders for alprazolam 0.5 mg to be delivered to the narcotics cart in various parts of the hospital on the following dates:
- February 1, 2011: dispensed100 tablets to the emergency room
- February 2, 2011: received 1000 tablets from wholesaler on invoice 0202201108
- February 2, 2011: dispensed 50 tablets to ICU
- February 3, 2011: received 10 outdated tablets from crash cart
- February 3, 2011: dispensed 30 tablets to crash cart
- February 4, 2011: dispensed 100 tablets to cardiac care unit
- February 5, 2011: dispensed 200 tablets to the emergency room

1. Based on the previous information, complete the following log.

Date	Dispensed	Received	Invoice Number	On-Hand Quantity
January 31, 2011	X	X	X	475

Lab Activity #10.3: Identify manufacturers of pharmacy automation using *www.rxinsider.com.*

Equipment needed:

- Computer with Internet connection
- Pencil/pen
- Paper

Time needed to complete this activity: 20 minutes

1. Identify five manufacturers of each of the following products/systems.

A. Automated Dispensing Cabinets

1. _____

2. _____

3. _____

4. _____

5. _____

B. Automation/Robotics

1. _____

2. _____

3. _____

4. _____

5. _____

C. Bar Code Supplies/Systems

1. _____
2. _____
3. _____
4. _____
5. _____

D. E-Prescribing Systems

1. _____
2. _____
3. _____
4. _____
5. _____

E. Hoods/Cleanrooms/Gloveboxes

1. _____
2. _____
3. _____
4. _____
5. _____

F. Pneumatic Tubes

1. _____
2. _____
3. _____
4. _____
5. _____

G. Tablet/Capsule Counters

1. _____
2. _____
3. _____
4. _____
5. _____

Lab Activity #10.4: Research automated dispensing systems

Equipment needed:

- Computer with Internet connection
- Computer printer
- Computer paper

Time needed to complete this activity: 45 minutes

Using the Internet, collect information about automated dispensing systems from the following websites:

- *www.*omnicell.com
- www.carefusion.com
- www.mckesson.com
- www.parata.com
- www.*swisslog.com*

1. Complete the following table.

Manufacturer	System	Features of the System	Benefits of the System
Omnicell	Pharmacy Workflow System		
	Controlled Substance Management		
	Medication Order Processing		
Pyxis	Pyxis Control Center		
	Pyxis Cubie System		
	Pyxis PARx System		
	Pyxis CII Safe		
	Pyxis Connect System		
	Pyxis Integrated Analytic Solutions		
	Pyxis Duo Station System		
	Pyxis MedStation System		
	Pyxis Remote Manager		
	Pyxis Specialty Station System		
McKesson	Fulfill-Rx		
	SKY Unit Dose Packing		
	Bar Code Medication Packaging Solution		
	PACMED		
	CPOE Solution		
Parata	Parata Max		
	Parata Mini		
Swisslog	ATP High-Speed Tablet Packager		
	PillPick		
	BoxPick		

11 Repackaging and Compounding

REINFORCE KEY CONCEPTS

TERMS AND DEFINITIONS

Select the correct term from the following list and write the corresponding letter in the blank next to the statement.

A. Blister packs
B. Bubble pack
C. Calibration
D. Compounding
E. Good manufacturing practice
F. Elixir
G. Granules
H. Hydrophilic
I. Hydrophobic
J. Mortar and pestle
K. Excipient
L. Reconstitution
M. Repackaging
N. Solute
O. Solution
P. Solvent
Q. Suspension
R. Syrup
S. Tincture
T. Aliquots
U. Triturate

___L___ 1. To mix a liquid and a powder to form a suspension or solution

___H___ 2. Water loving; any substance that easily dissolves in water

___Q___ 3. A solution in which solid particles do not dissolve into the base, requiring the solution to be shaken before use

___D___ 4. The act of mixing, reconstituting, and packaging a drug

___A___ 5. Pre-formed card with transparent depressions that hold medications, sealed with a foil backboard

___U___ 6. To grind or crush powder such as a tablet into fine particles

___J___ 7. A bowl and rounded knob used to grind substances into fine powder

___M___ 8. The act of reducing the amount of medication taken from a bulk bottle; unit dosing

T ___~~T~~ ~~K~~___ 9. Part or portion of a medicine and/or ingredient that has the same volume or weight

___F___ 10. A base solution that is a mixture of alcohol and water

___N___ 11. The ingredient that is dissolved into a solution

___R___ 12. A sugar-based liquid

G ___~~X~~___ 13. Small particle or grain of individual ingredients or the entire composition of the agent

___B___ 14. Containers, usually made of plastic, that hold a single dose tablet or capsule

___S___ 15. A base solution of alcohol

C ___~~X~~ ~~G~~___ 16. The markings on a measuring device

___O___ 17. A water base in which the ingredients dissolve completely

___E___ 18. Federal guidelines that must be followed by all entities that prepare and package medication or medical devices

___I___ 19. Water hating; any substance that does not dissolve in water

___P___ 20. The greater part of a solution

K ___~~X~~ ~~T~~___ 21. Inert substance added to a drug to form a suitable consistency for dosing

TRUE OR FALSE

Write T or F next to each statement.

___T___ 1. Repackaging of medication is a common process in a hospital pharmacy.

___F___ 2. No expiration date is necessary for repackaged products.

___F___ 3. The process of repackaging should be done in a horizontal flow hood.

___T___ 4. If the expiration date includes the month and year, the drug expires on the first day of the month.

___T___ 5. Part of the preparation for repackaging is accurate calculations.

___F___ 6. Jars and syringes are the only packages that do not have childproof caps or lids.

___F___ 7. All records are to be kept in the pharmacy for only 1 year from the time the medication was prepared.

___T___ 8. The record-keeping part of compounding is extremely important.

___F___ 9. Capsule size 000 is the smallest size.

___T___ 10. Graduated cylinders are available in conical and cylindrical shapes.

MULTIPLE CHOICE

Complete each question by circling the best answer.

1. Which of the following is *not* a reason the pharmacy repackages a bulk drug into unit dose?
   A. The cost is lower when this process is done by the hospital
   B. Manufacturers do not package the drug in unit dose
   C. Unit dose medications can be recycled and used on another patient
   D. Unit dose is easier to count

2. The dosage form normally repackaged in a pharmacy is the:
   A. Tablet form
   B. Capsule form
   C. Liquid form
   D. All of the above

3. The expiration date on a drug is 2/07; the drug expires on:
   A. The first day of February 2007
   B. The last day of February 2007
   C. The first day of July 2002
   D. The last day of July 2002

4. The most common nonsterile, repackaged items in a hospital are:
   A. Creams, ointments, and oral suspensions
   B. Tablets, capsules, and liquids (solutions and suspensions)
   C. All of the above
   D. None of the above

5. A factor that can affect the stability of a drug is:
   A. Light
   B. Air
   C. Temperature
   D. All of the above

6. The punch method is used to prepare:

  A. Solutions

  B. Tablets

  C. Capsules

  D. Ointments

7. Good manufacturing practices do not include which of the following?

  A. Equipment in good and clean condition

  B. Medications checked by a technician

  C. Appropriate packaging for the drugs

  D. Records logged for referencing

8. A class _____ balance weighs _____ substances, and a class _____ balance weighs _____ substances.

  A. A, lighter; B, heavier

  B. A, heavier; B, lighter

  C. A, both heavy and light; B, both heavy and light

  D. A, both heavy and light, B, light

MATCHING

Matching I

Match the following terms with their meanings.

_____ B _____ 1. Unit dose

_____ D _____ 2. Monthly supply

_____ E _____ 3. Recipe book

_____ A _____ 4. Dosage form

_____ C _____ 5. Mortar and pestle

A. Tablet, capsule, spansule
B. One medication dose per container
C. Compounding equipment
D. 30-Day supply
E. Formula cards

Matching II

Match the following dosage forms with their auxiliary labels.

_____ D _____ 1. Ophthalmics

_____ E _____ 2. Otics

_____ A _____ 3. Ointments, creams, lotions

_____ C _____ 4. Suppositories

_____ B _____ 5. Patches

A. For topical use; external use
B. Apply to skin
C. For rectal use
D. For the eye
E. For the ear

FILL IN THE BLANK

Answer each question by completing the statement in the space provided.

1. What auxiliary label is used with oral suspensions? _____

2. The base ingredient of a suppository is usually a combination of _____ and _____.

3. You must have liquids at _____ level to read the bottom of the liquid line, known as the

    _____.

4. To prepare an ointment, a _____ base must be mixed with the drug. To prepare a cream, a

    _____ base is used.

5. What type of compounding equipment is used to weigh powders? _____

6. A _____ and _____ are used to crush tablets and other solid substances.

7. Name three additional ingredients used to reduce the bad taste of drugs.

    A. _____

    B. _____

    C. _____

SHORT ANSWER

Write a short response to each question in the space provided.

1. Why is it necessary to use tweezers to grasp metal weights?

    _____

    _____

2. Why is it necessary to clean counting trays?

    _____

    _____

RESEARCH ACTIVITY

Follow the instructions given in each exercise and provide a response.

Access the following compounding websites:

- *www.pccarx.com*
- *www.pharmacytimes.com/compounding*

1. What types of services do they provide?

2. Find an interesting compounding recipe (if published). Print it and share it with the class.

3. Is membership required to use these sites and to obtain their products?

CRITICAL THINKING

Reply to each question based on what you have learned in the chapter.

1. Pediatric medications sometimes require special compounding. What are some ways the pharmacy staff can accommodate pediatric patients to foster their compliance in taking their medications?

   we can add sugar excipients to make it more flavorful and/or color additives to make it more aesthetically pleasing to the child's eye.

2. Preparing capsules using the punch method can be messy. What techniques for preparing capsules can you develop to minimize the mess?

   Be very organized and thorough. Have good technique when holding capsule so you do not spill or knock powder. Be calm and collected and make sure you have all of the powder in the capsule.

3. Mrs. Foster has been coming to your pharmacy for years. Lately, she has become hard of hearing and often misinterprets the pharmacist's directions about her medications.
   A. How can you, as a technician, aid in this process?

   Do not rely on her hearing for understanding directions. Put it in writing for her. Let the pharmacist know she is hard of hearing and has difficulty understanding directions.

   B. What tools can you develop to help Mrs. Foster understand how to take her medications?

   Have good penmanship and make sure she wants to be counseled before involving the pharmacist. Have compassion for her and her situation.

151

LAB SCENARIOS

Pharmacy Equipment Used in Compounding Nonsterile Preparations

Objective: To introduce the pharmacy technician to the equipment used in preparing nonsterile preparations.

Lab Activity #11.1: Correctly identify the following pharmacy equipment used in extemporaneous compounding and its purpose.

Equipment needed:

- Beaker
- Compounding record
- Conical graduate
- Counterbalance
- Cylindrical graduate
- Droppers
- Electronic scale
- Erlenmeyer flask
- Filter paper
- Forceps
- Funnel
- Glacine paper
- Glass funnel
- Glass mortar and pestle
- Hot plate
- Latex gloves
- Masks
- Metric weights
- Ointment slab
- Parchment paper
- Pipette
- Porcelain mortar and pestle
- Reconstitution tube
- Rubber spatula
- Safety glass
- Stainless steel spatula
- Stirring rod
- Suppository molds
- Tongs
- Torsion balance
- Wedgwood mortar and pestle
- Weighing boat

Time needed to complete this activity: 20 minutes

Equipment	Correctly Identified (Yes/No)	Purpose
Beaker		
Compounding record		
Conical graduate		
Cylindrical graduate		
Counterbalance		
Dropper		
Electronic scale		
Erlenmeyer flask		
Filter paper		
Forceps		
Funnel		
Glacine paper		
Glass funnel		
Glass mortar and pestle		
Hot plate		
Latex gloves		
Masks		
Metric weights		
Ointment slab		
Parchment papers		
Pipette		
Pipette filler		
Porcelain mortar and pestle		
Reconstitution tube		
Rubber spatula		
Safety glasses		
Stainless steel spatula		
Stirring rod		
Suppository molds		
Tongs		
Torsion balance		
Wedgwood mortar and pestle		
Weighing boat		

Chapter **11** **Repackaging and Compounding**

Lab Activity #11.2: Define the following terms used in nonsterile compounding.

Equipment needed:

- Medical dictionary
- Pencil/pen

Time needed to complete this activity: 15 minutes

1. Blending

_____

2. Comminution

_____

3. Diluent

_____

4. Geometric dilution

_____

5. Inert substance

_____

6. Levigation

_____

7. Pulverization

_____

8. Punch method

_____

9. Sifting

_____

10. Solvent

_____

11. Spatulation

_____

12. Trituration

_____

13. Tumbling

_____

The Class A Scale and Weighing Ingredients

Objective: Demonstrate proper procedures in weighing solids in the practice of pharmacy.

Weighing refers to the determination of a definite weight of a material to be used in the compounding of a prescription or the manufacturing of a dosage form. Weight is measured by means of a balance. Four types of balances are used in pharmacy practice: single beam (equal-arm or unequal), compound lever, torsion, and electronic. All pharmacies are required to have a Class A (III) balance, which can be a torsion balance. An unequal arm balance is used to measure weights greater than 60 grams and is commonly used in manufacturing.

A torsion balance must have a maximum sensitivity of 6 milligrams with no load, and with full load to one pan must cause the indicator or the rest point to be shifted not less than one division on the index point. A torsion balance can weigh up to 60 grams. An electronic balance has a sensitivity of less than 10 mg and can weigh quantities of a drug more accurately than a torsion balance.

If a pharmacy uses a torsion balance, it must have a set of metric weights that consists of one 50-g, two 20-g, one 10-g, one 5-g, two-2 g, one 1-g, one 500-mg, two-200 mg, one 100-mg, one 50-mg, two 20-mg, and one 10-mg weight. These weights are made of brass, and forceps must be used in placing the weight on the pan.

Lab Activity #11.3: Identify the following components of a Class A prescription balance.

Equipment needed:

- Class A balance

Time needed to complete this activity: 5 minutes

Identifying the Parts of a Class A Balance Evaluation	Yes/No	Purpose
Calibrated dial		
Graduate dial		
Index plate		
Leveling screw feet		
Locking or arrest arm		
Weighing pans		

Lab Activity #11.4: Calibrating a Class A prescription balance

Equipment needed:

- Class A prescription balance

Procedure

1. Arrest the balance by turning the arrest arm.
2. Level the balance from front to back by turning the leveling screw feet. Move leveling screw feet until all four sides of the balance are at the same distance from the surface on which they are resting.
3. Turn the calibrated dial to zero.
4. Level balance from left to right by adjusting the leveling screw feet.

Time needed to complete this activity: 5 minutes

Calibrating a Class A Balance Evaluation	Yes/No
"Arresting" the balance	
Leveling the balance	
Balance calibrated to zero	
Level the balance	

Lab Activity #11.5: Using a torsion or electronic balance to weigh the proper quantity of ingredient

Equipment needed:

- Disinfecting agent/cleanser
- Forceps
- Latex gloves
- Lint-free paper towels
- Metal spatula
- Metric weights
- Sink with running hot and cold water
- Solid powder such as flour or sugar
- Torsion balance
- Weighing boats or glacine paper

Procedure

1. Wash hands and put on latex gloves.
2. Calibrate the Class A balance.
3. Lock balance.
4. Place a weighing boat or glacine paper on each pan.
5. Unlock the balance by releasing the arrest knob.
6. Make sure the pointer is resting at the center of the index.
7. Arrest the balance.
8. Place the correct weights on the right pan by using forceps.
9. Place the material to be weighed on the left pan using a spatula.
10. Release the balance.
11. If the pointer moves to the left, there is too much ingredient on the left pan. If the pointer moves to the right, there is not enough ingredient on the left pan.
12. Remove or add ingredient by using the spatula. Arrest the balance each time before material is added or released.
13. Double-check that the amount weighed on the left pan is correct.

Time needed to complete this activity: 20 minutes

Weight	Amount Weighed
20 mg	
65 mg	
83 mg	
554 mg	
858 mg	
1.25 g	
10 g	
21.25 g	
28.37 g	
45.3 g	

Measuring Liquids

Objective: Demonstrate the proper procedures in measuring liquids in the practice of pharmacy.

Measuring refers to the exact determination of a definite volume of liquid. Glass measures are preferred for measuring liquids because they can indicate volume more accurately by the transparency of the glass.

When an aqueous or alcoholic liquid is poured into a graduate, surface forces cause its surface to become concave—the portion in contact with the liquid is drawn upward resulting in the formation of a meniscus. Two types of graduates are available: cylindrical and conical. The conical graduate is suitable for some measurements, but cylindrical graduates are more accurate because of their uniform and smaller average diameter. Pipettes are more accurate and convenient than very small graduates in measuring very small volumes. The very narrow bore permits greater distances between graduations on the apparatus, thus allowing greater accuracy in making the reading.

Lab Activity #11.6: Using a graduate cylinder of correct size, measure the following volumes and indicate the volume of the graduate cylinder that was used and why it was selected.

Procedure

1. Wash hands and put on latex gloves.
2. Select a graduate of proper size; the selected graduate should not measure less than 20% of the capacity of the graduate.
3. Hold the graduate in the left hand and grasp the original container with the label in such apposition that any excess of liquid will not soil the label if it should run down the container.
4. Raise the graduate and hold it at eye level, so that the graduation point to be read is level with the eye, and measure the liquid.
5. Pour the liquid slowly into the graduate.
6. Remove excess liquid or add additional liquid to measure the proper quantity of liquid.

Equipment needed:

- Disinfecting agent/cleanser
- Graduate cylinder 10 ml
- Latex gloves
- Lint-free paper towels
- Sink with running hot and cold water
- Water

Time needed to complete this activity: 15 minutes

Volume	Amount Measured	Size of Graduate Cylinder Used	Reason for Selection of Graduate
2.5 ml			
5 ml			
9 ml			
10 ml			
24 ml			
30 ml			
38 ml			
48 ml			
66 ml			
88 ml			

Lab Activity #11.7: Measuring a liquid using a pipette

Equipment needed:

- Disinfecting agent/cleanser
- Empty containers (2)
- Latex gloves
- Lint-free paper towels
- Pipette
- Pipette filler
- Sink with running hot and cold water
- Water

Procedure

1. Wash hands and put on latex gloves.
2. Insert the pipette into the liquid to be withdrawn.
3. Squeeze the pipette bulb slowly.
4. Gently release your grip until the correct amount is withdrawn.
5. Remove the pipette from the liquid and hold above the container to which the liquid is being removed.
6. Remove the bulb while holding your finger over the top of the pipette, slowly allowing the correct amount of liquid to flow into the empty container by releasing your finger from the top of the pipette.

Measuring a Liquid Using a Pipette Evaluation	Yes/No
¼ of a pipette	
½ of a pipette	
¾ of a pipette	
1 pipette	

Preparing Powders and Capsules

Objective: Demonstrate proper techniques in preparing capsules by using the punch method. Complete a compounding log, and assign the correct beyond-use date.

A powder is a solid dosage form that can be taken orally and externally, depending on the drug being used. Powders are used in compounding tablets, capsules, and suspensions. A capsule is a solid dosage form in which the drug substance is enclosed in a hard or soft, soluble container or shell of a suitable form of gelatin. A hard gelatin capsule, also known as a dry-filled capsule, consists of two sections. These capsules range in size from 000 to 5, measuring from 600 to 30 mg. A soft elastic capsule is a soft, globular gelatin shell somewhat thicker than that of a hard gelatin capsule. A capsule dissolves in the stomach after 10 to 30 minutes, and the drug is released. A capsule eliminates objectionable tastes and odors of certain drugs.

A compounding log or mixing record is an official detailed record of the processes and materials used in the compounding process. A compounding log contains the name of the final product; the quantity prepared; a copy of the patient label; the recipe; the names, lot numbers, and quantities of all products and ingredients used; a record of the steps followed to prepare the prescription; the lot number assigned to the final product; and a beyond-use date.

Manufactured drug products are assigned an expiration date for the drug product. USP 795 (nonsterile preparations) requires that all compounded products have beyond-use dating. Under USP 795, a refrigerated aqueous solution has a beyond-use date of 14 days, and for a nonaqueous liquid or solid formulation (for which the manufactured drug product is the source of the active ingredient), the beyond-use date is not later than 25% of the time remaining until the expiration date, or 6 months, whichever is earlier. If a USP or NF substance is the source of the active ingredient, the beyond-use date is not later than 6 months. For all other formulations, the beyond-use date is not later than the intended duration of therapy, or 30 days, whichever is earlier.

Lab Activity #11.8: Preparing powders

Equipment needed:

- Class A balance
- Disinfecting agent/cleanser
- Latex gloves
- Lint-free paper towels
- Mortar and pestle
- Powder papers
- Sieve
- Sink with running hot and cold water
- Spatula
- Powder A
- Powder B
- Powder C
- Weighing boats

Procedure

1. Collect the appropriate equipment and supplies for this procedure.
2. Wash hands properly and place gloves on hands.
3. Triturate (grind) each powder using the correct mortar and pestle in a circular motion to reduce the particle size of each powder. Begin with the ingredient with the smallest quantity.

4. Continue the trituration process by adding the next smallest quantity of powder to the previously triturated powder. This process is known as geometric dilution.
5. Add the last powder to the mortar containing the two previously triturated products, and repeat the process.
6. Blend (mix) all three powders until the particle size is uniform and the powders are mixed thoroughly.
7. Stir the powder thoroughly using the appropriate spatula.
8. Pour the mixed powders through a sieve to a compounding slab.
9. Tare the torsion balance and place weighing boats on each side.
10. Weigh the correct quantity of powder.
11. Empty the ingredients from the weighing boat into a powder paper.
12. Fold powder paper.
13. Complete compounding log.

Time to needed complete this activity: 20 minutes

Pharmacy Compounding Log						
Drug Name	Lot Number	Mfg. Expiration Date	Quantity Prepared	Measured by	Verified by	Beyond-Use Date

Compounding Powder Evaluation	Yes/No
Proper equipment and materials selected	
Washed hands properly and put on latex gloves	
Powder #1 triturated properly	
Powder #2 triturated properly	
Powder #3 triturated properly	
Powders added in correct order	
Powder blended properly	
Stirred powders properly with a spatula	
Sifted powders properly	
Weighed the proper quantity of powder for each powder paper	
Poured powder into papers and folded properly to avoid spillage	
Completed compounding record	

Lab Activity #11.9: Compounding capsules

Equipment needed:

- 10 acetaminophen 500-mg tablets
- 10 empty size 0 gelatin capsules
- Clean gauze
- Counting tray
- Disinfecting agent/cleanser
- Electronic or torsion balance
- Latex gloves
- Lint-free paper towels
- Metal spatula
- Ointment slab
- Sink with running hot and cold water

- Soap
- Wedgewood mortar and pestle
- Weighing boat or glacine paper

Procedure

1. Gather supplies necessary for this exercise.
2. Wash hands thoroughly and put on latex gloves.
3. Count out 10 acetaminophen 500-mg tablets in a counting tray.
4. Pour tablets into a Wedgwood mortar. Triturate with Wedgwood pestle.
5. Pour acetaminophen powder from mortar onto ointment slab.
6. Scrape remaining acetaminophen from mortar with spatula onto ointment slab.
7. Remove the capsule cap from the capsule body.
8. Take the body of the capsule, open side down with thumb and first finger.
9. Punch capsule into acetaminophen powder. After reaching the bottom of the powder on the ointment slab, turn capsule lightly and pinch the open end of the capsule.
10. Repeat the process with the same capsule until body of capsule is filled.
11. Place the capsule cap on the body of the capsule.
12. Place torsion or electronic balance on flat surface; turn it on and allow it to go to "0."
13. Place an empty capsule in weighing boat or on glacine paper, and obtain reading.
14. Press the "tare" button to reset the scale to zero.
15. Remove empty capsule from weighing boat.
16. Place the filled capsule on the weighing boat and weigh the capsule.
17. If the capsule weighs more than 500 mg, gently remove the cap from the body of the capsule and take out some of the powder from the capsule; reweigh the capsule. If the capsule weighs less than 500 mg, remove the cap from the body of the capsule, add powder from the ointment slab, and reweigh the filled capsule.
18. Wipe off powder from exterior of capsule with a dry piece of gauze.
19. Repeat this process four additional times and record the weight of each capsule in the table below.
20. Complete the compounding record.

Time to needed complete this activity: 30 minutes

Capsule #	Desired Weight	Actual Weight	Difference
1	500 mg		
2	500 mg		
3	500 mg		
4	500 mg		
5	500 mg		
6	500 mg		
7	500 mg		
8	500 mg		
9	500 mg		

Pharmacy Compounding Log						
Drug Name	Lot Number	Mfg. Expiration Date	Quantity Prepared	Measured by	Verified by	Beyond-Use Date

Evaluation of Capsule Preparation	Yes/No
Washed hands properly and put on latex gloves	
Counted out proper quantity of tablets	
Selected correct mortar and pestle	
Triturated tablets to a fine powder	
Filled capsules properly	
Balance tared	
Final weight of capsules within 2 mg of desired weight	
Excess powder removed from exterior of capsule	
Compounding log filled out	
Correct beyond-use date assigned	

Reconstituting a Solid

Objective: Demonstrate the proper steps in reconstituting a powder into a solution.

Reconstitution is the process by which a predetermined quantity of liquid is added to a powder to form a solution or a suspension. The drug manufacturer provides on the drug label the quantity and type of liquid to be added to the powder.

Lab Activity #11.10: Reconstituting a solid

Equipment needed:

- "Shake well" label
- 6 fl oz amber bottle
- Disinfecting agent/cleanser
- Distilled water
- Electronic or torsion balance
- Lint-free paper towels
- Reconstitution tube
- Sink with running hot and cold water
- Steel spatula
- Sugar
- Weighing boat/glacine paper

Procedure

1. Gather supplies necessary for this exercise.
2. Wash hands thoroughly and put on latex gloves.
3. Measure 2 g of sugar and pour into 6 fl oz amber bottle.
4. Bring amber bottle with sugar in it to reconstitution area.
5. Make sure the lower clamp on the reconstitution tube is clamped closed by pinching the clamp until it clicks shut.
6. Open the upper clamp on the reconstitution tube by clicking the clamp open.
7. Allow 88 ml of distilled water to flow into the reconstitution tube. When the tube is filled to 88 ml, close the upper clamp by pinching it shut.
8. Shake the amber bottle to loosen the sugar, and remove the bottle top.
9. Place the tip of the lower tube of reconstitution tube into mouth of amber bottle.
10. Open the lower clamp to allow approximately ⅔ of the water (60 ml) to enter the amber bottle slowly. Close lower clamp.
11. Place bottle top back on bottle and shake amber bottle with distilled water-sugar solution until solution is evenly dissolved.

Chapter **11** **Repackaging and Compounding**

12. Remove bottle top and place the reconstitution tube into the mouth of the amber bottle; add remaining water from reconstitution tube into amber bottle and shake well.
13. Tightly recap the amber bottle and shake thoroughly.
14. Complete the compounding log.

Time needed to complete this activity: 10 minutes

Pharmacy Compounding Log						
Drug Name	Lot Number	Mfg. Expiration Date	Quantity Prepared	Measured by	Verified by	Beyond-Use Date

Reconstituting a Solid Powder Evaluation	Yes/No
Gathered equipment and supplies	
Washed hands properly and put on latex gloves	
Electronic or torsion balance tared	
2 g of sugar weighed properly	
Sugar transferred to amber bottle	
88 ml of distilled water measured properly in reconstitution tube	
⅔ of water emptied from reconstitution tube into amber bottle with sugar	
Remaining water from reconstitution tube emptied into amber bottle with sugar solution	
Affixed "Shake well" label to amber bottle	
Compounding log filled out	
Correct beyond-use date assigned	

Nonsterile Compounding of Syrups and Elixirs

Objective: Demonstrate the proper technique in preparing an oral syrup.

A syrup is a concentrated, viscous, aqueous solution of sugar or sugar substitute with or without flavors and medical substances. When purified water alone is used in making the solution of sucrose, the preparation is known as a syrup or simple syrup if the sucrose concentration is 85%. Sometimes alcohol is included in the preparation of syrup as a preservative and a solvent for flavors. A medicated syrup is one that contains a medicinal syrup. A flavored syrup is not usually medicated and is intended as a vehicle or flavor for prescriptions.

Syrups possess the ability to mask the taste of bitter or saline drugs. Disadvantages of syrups include the possibility of producing cavities and gingivitis in individuals. Another concern regarding syrups is the calorie content due to sugar.

Syrups can be compounded by using one of the following four techniques: solution with heat, solution by agitation, addition of sucrose to a liquid medication or flavored vehicle, and percolation. Solution with heat can be used if the ingredients are not volatile or can be broken down by heat. Purified water is heated to 80 to 85° C; it is removed from its source of heat and sucrose is added. Other ingredients can be added at this time, and the solution is able to cool down. Agitation without heat is used when heat would cause the ingredients to break down. During this process, sugar is dissolved in purified water in a container that is larger than the volume being prepared and is shaken vigorously. Addition of sucrose to a liquid medication or a flavored extract is often used with fluid extracts and tinctures. A disadvantage of this process is that a precipitant may develop. Percolation is the process by which purified water is passed slowly over a bed of crystalline sugar, resulting in a syrup.

An elixir is a clear, pleasantly flavored, sweetened hydroalcoholic liquid for oral use. The primary ingredients in an elixir are ethanol and water, but glycerin, sorbitol, propylene glycol flavoring agents, preservatives, and syrups are also used. An elixir is more fluid than syrup and uses less sucrose than syrup. An elixir can be used as a vehicle for flavors and medications. An elixir does not mask the taste of saline ingredients. A major disadvantage of elixirs is their many incompatibilities with medications.

Lab Activity #11.11: Compounding syrup-NF

Equipment needed:

- Beaker
- Disinfecting agent/cleanser
- 4-ounce prescription bottle
- Graduate cylinder
- Latex gloves
- Lint-free paper towels
- Metric weights
- Purified water
- Sink with running hot and cold water
- Sucrose
- Torsion or electronic balance

Procedure

1. Organize materials on workbench.
2. Wash hands and dry thoroughly.
3. Place gloves on hands.
4. Tare torsion or electronic balance.
5. Place weighing boat on balance.
6. Weigh 85 g of sucrose and place in a beaker that has a capacity greater than 100 ml.
7. Measure 100 ml of purified water in graduate cylinder.
8. Add purified water to sucrose.
9. Agitate (shake) sucrose solution slowly.
10. Pour sucrose solution into a 4-ounce bottle and qs up to 100 ml.
11. Label as Simple Syrup 100 ml.
12. Complete the compounding log.
13. Clean equipment.

Time needed to complete this activity: 20 minutes

Pharmacy Compounding Log						
Drug Name	Lot Number	Mfg. Expiration Date	Quantity Prepared	Measured by	Verified by	Beyond-Use Date

Compounding a Syrup Evaluation	Yes/No
Materials organized	
Hands washed properly and dried	
Latex gloves on hands	
Balance tared	
Sucrose weighed properly	
Purified water measured properly	
Ingredients added properly	
Sucrose solution thoroughly shaken	
Sucrose solution poured into prescription bottle of proper size	
Syrup qs to 100 ml with purified water	
Labeled	
Compounding log completed	
Cleaned equipment	

Lab Activity #11.12: Compounding an elixir

Prepare 4 fluid ounces of acetaminophen elixir using the following formula:

Acetaminophen	4.0 g
Propylene glycol	50 ml
Ethanol	200 ml
Sorbitol solution	600 ml
Saccharin sodium	5.0 g
Flavor	qs
Purified water, to make	1000 ml

Equipment needed:

- Acetaminophen tablets
- Calculator
- Disinfecting agent/cleanser
- Ethanol
- Filter paper
- 4-ounce prescription bottle
- Funnel
- Graduate cylinders
- Latex gloves
- Lint-free paper towels
- Propylene glycol
- Purified water
- Saccharin sodium
- Sink with running hot and cold water
- Sorbitol solution
- Spatula
- Torsion or electronic balance
- Wedgwood mortar and pestle
- Weighing boat

Procedure

1. Perform the necessary calculations using a calculator to reduce the formula to 120 ml.
2. Organize materials on workbench.
3. Wash hands and dry thoroughly.
4. Place gloves on hands.
5. Count out the correct number of acetaminophen tablets/geltabs.
6. Triturate acetaminophen tablets/geltabs.
7. Tare torsion or electronic balance.
8. Count out the correct quantity of saccharin sodium tablets.
9. Triturate the saccharin sodium tablets.
10. Weigh correct amount of triturated acetaminophen in weighing boat on balance.
11. Weigh correct amount of saccharin sodium in weighing boat on balance.
12. Measure the proper volumes of sorbitol solution, ethanol, and purified water in graduate cylinders.
13. Dissolve water-soluble ingredients in part of water.
14. Add and solubilize the sucrose in the aqueous solution.
15. Prepare an alcoholic solution containing the other ingredients.
16. Add the aqueous phase to the alcoholic solution.
17. Fold filter paper and place in funnel on top graduate cylinder.
18. Filter the elixir.
19. Qs the elixir to 120 ml with purified water.
20. Transfer elixir to 4-ounce prescription bottle.
21. Label.
22. Complete compounding log.
23. Clean equipment and put away.

164

Time needed to complete this activity: 30 minutes

Pharmacy Compounding Log						
Drug Name	Lot Number	Mfg. Expiration Date	Quantity Prepared	Measured by	Verified by	Beyond-Use Date

Compounding an Elixir Evaluation	Yes/No
Reduced formula to 120 ml	
Materials organized	
Hands washed and dried	
Gloves on hands	
Correct quantities of acetaminophen and saccharin tablets	
Acetaminophen triturated	
Saccharin triturated	
Liquids measured properly in correct graduates	
Water-soluble ingredients dissolved in water	
Sucrose mixed in aqueous phase	
Alcoholic solution prepared	
Aqueous solution added to alcoholic solution	
Elixir filtered	
Transferred elixir to prescription bottle of proper size	
Labeled	
Compounding log completed	
Equipment cleaned and put away	

Nonsterile Compounding of Suspensions

Objective: Demonstrate the proper technique in preparing a suspension.

A suspension is a coarse dispersion containing finely divided insoluble material suspended in a liquid. All suspensions require that a suspending agent be used in their preparation. Examples of suspending agents include Avicel, Methocel, Metocel, Tylopur, Culminol, Celocel, Ethicel, Natrasol, Cellocize, Bermacol, Tylose, Carbopol, Povidone, and Kollidon. Sometimes a product can be prepared in dry form and is placed in the form of a suspension, with water added at the time of dispensing. A suspension may be taken orally, injected intramuscularly or subcutaneously, instilled intranasally, inhaled into the lungs, applied as a topical preparation, or used as an ophthalmic agent. Suspensions offer the following advantages over other dosage forms:

- They offer an alternative oral dosage form for patients who are unable to swallow a tablet or capsule, especially pediatric and geriatric patients.
- Some medications are poorly water soluble and cannot be formulated as solutions.
- Some drugs have an unpleasant taste, and a suspension allows for less interaction with the taste receptors in the mouth.
- Suspensions offer a method to provide sustained release of a drug by parenteral, topical, and oral routes of administration.

It is important to remember the size of the dispersed particles so they do not settle rapidly in their container. However, if the particles do settle in the container, they should be able to be redispersed with minimum effort by the patient. In addition, the suspension should be easy to pour, should have a pleasant taste, and should be resistant to microbial attack.

Chapter **11** **Repackaging and Compounding**

Lab Activity #11.13: Compounding a suspension

Equipment needed:
- "Shake well" label
- Acetaminophen, 24 500 mg tablets or caplets
- Class A balance
- Disinfecting agent/cleanser
- Graduate
- Latex gloves
- Light-resistant bottle
- Lint-free paper towels
- Mortar and pestle
- Sink with running hot and cold water
- Size 100 sieve
- Spatula
- Stirring rod
- 120 ml of Syrpalta (or other wetting agent)

Procedure

1. Organize supplies on workbench.
2. Wash hands thoroughly.
3. Weigh the dry ingredients.
4. Triturate all dry ingredients with a mortar and pestle.
5. Filter a pulverized powder through a size 100 mesh sieve.
6. Measure 120 ml of Syrpalta into a graduate cylinder.
7. Wet the powder with Syrpalta in the mortar.
8. Stir while continuing to add Syrpalta until it forms a thick paste.
9. Pour the mixture into a graduate.
10. Add the remaining Syrpalta until the desired volume is obtained.
11. Stir mixture until it is mixed thoroughly.
12. Pour suspension into a container of appropriate size.
13. Label suspension properly.
14. Complete the compounding log.
15. Clean equipment.

Time to needed complete this activity: 20 minutes

Pharmacy Compounding Log						
Drug Name	Lot Number	Mfg. Expiration Date	Quantity Prepared	Measured by	Verified by	Beyond-Use Date

Compounding a Suspension Evaluation	Yes/No
Materials organized	
Hands washed	
Counted out the correct quantity of tablets or caplets of acetaminophen	
Measured Syrpalta correctly	
Triturated ingredients properly	
Filtered powder with sieve	
Added Syrpalta	
QS pasted to proper volume	
Suspension properly mixed	
Poured suspension into container of proper size	
Labeled correctly	
Compounding log completed	

Nonsterile Compounding of Emulsions

Objective: Demonstrate the proper technique in preparing an emulsion.

An emulsion is a dispersed system containing at least two immiscible liquid phases. An emulsion consists of at least three components: the dispersed phase, the dispersion medium, and an emulsifying agent. One of the two immiscible liquids is aqueous, and the second is oil. The emulsifying agent used and the quantities of aqueous and oil phases will determine whether the emulsion is oil-in-water (O/W) or water-in-oil (W/O). An oil-in-water emulsion finds oil dispersed as droplets in the aqueous phase. Conversely, when water is dispersed in the oil phase, it is known as a water-in-oil emulsion. Oral emulsions are normally oil-in-water; emulsified lotions may be O/W or W/O, depending on their usage.

Two distinct processes occur in the preparation of an emulsion. Flocculation is the process of clumping together particles or drops. Meanwhile, coalescence occurs when two immiscible liquids are shaken together. An emulsifying agent reduces the possibility that coalescence may occur. An emulsifying agent should
- Be able reduce surface tension
- Absorb quickly around the dispersed drops, which will prevent the drops from coalescing
- Provide an electrical potential, so drops repel each other
- Increase the viscosity of the emulsion
- Be effective in low concentration

Emulsifying agents may be classified as synthetic, natural, or finely divided. Examples of emulsifying agents include potassium laureate, triethanolamine stearate, sodium lauryl sulfate, dioctyl sodium sulfosuccinate, acacia, gelatin, lecithin, cholesterol, and bentonite. In some situations, multiple emulsifying agents may be used in the preparation of an emulsion.

Lab Activity #11.14: Compounding an emulsion using the dry gum method

Equipment needed:
- Active ingredients
- Class A balance
- Disinfecting agent/cleanser
- Graduate
- Gum acacia
- Label
- Latex gloves
- Light-resistant container
- Lint-free paper towels
- Mortar and pestle
- Oil
- Sink with running hot and cold water
- Spatula
- Water
- Weighing boats

Procedure

1. Gather all equipment and materials.
2. Wash hands thoroughly
3. Measure oil and pour the oil into the mortar.
4. Place the desired amount of gum acacia into the mortar.
5. Triturate until the acacia is thoroughly wet and smooth.
6. Measure the appropriate amount of water desired for the aqueous phase in a clean graduate.
7. Triturate the mixture with a firm motion and quick movement until the primary emulsion is formed. The emulsion will change from a transparent liquid to a white liquid. The sound associated with the trituration process will change.
8. Add the remaining ingredients until the final volume is reached.
9. Homogenize the emulsion.
10. Pour into a container of appropriate size.
11. Label the container.
12. Complete the compounding log.
13. Clean equipment.

Time to needed complete this activity: 20 minutes

Pharmacy Compounding Log

Drug Name	Lot Number	Mfg. Expiration Date	Quantity Prepared	Measured by	Verified by	Beyond-Use Date

Compounding an Emulsion (Dry Gum Method) Evaluation	Yes/No
Hands washed	
Oil measured properly and poured into the proper mortar	
Weighed the correct amount of acacia and poured into mortar	
Triturated acacia properly	
Measured water properly in the correct graduate	
Triturated oil-acacia-water mixture properly	
Mixture qs to proper volume	
Poured emulsion into bottle of proper size	
Bottle labeled correctly	
Compound log completed	

Lab Activity #11.15: Compounding an emulsion using the wet gum method

Equipment needed:
- Active ingredients
- Disinfecting agent/cleanser
- Glycerin
- Graduate
- Gum acacia
- Label
- Latex gloves
- Light-resistant container
- Lint-free paper towels
- Oil
- Sink with running hot and cold water
- Syrup
- Water
- Wedgwood mortar and pestle

Procedure

1. Gather all equipment and materials.
2. Wash hands thoroughly.
3. Place the desired amount of gum acacia into a Wedgwood mortar.
4. Slowly add the desired amount of water while triturating the mixture.
5. Gradually add the correct volume of oil while triturating the mixture.
6. Measure syrup and weigh active ingredient.
7. Add remaining ingredients to mixture and qs to proper volume.
8. Pour mixture into container of proper size.
9. Label container properly.
10. Complete compounding log.

Time needed to complete this activity: 20 minutes

Pharmacy Compounding Log						
Drug Name	**Lot Number**	**Mfg. Expiration Date**	**Quantity Prepared**	**Measured by**	**Verified by**	**Beyond-Use Date**

Compounding an Emulsion (Wert Gum Method) Evaluation	Yes/No
Hands washed	
Acacia weighed correctly and poured into correct mortar and pestle	
Water measured in correct graduate	
Water poured into mixture and triturated	
Oil measured, poured into mixture, and triturated	
Syrup measured correctly	
Active ingredient weighed properly	
Emulsion poured into container of proper size	
Container labeled correctly	
Compounding record completed properly	

Nonsterile Compounding of Creams and Ointments

Objective: Demonstrate the proper technique in preparing an ointment.

An ointment is a semisolid preparation intended for external application to the skin or mucous membranes. Normally, it contains a medication. Four different types of bases are used in the preparation of an ointment: hydrocarbon (oleaginous), absorption, water removable (water washable), and water washable bases.

A hydrocarbon base is selected when the ointment will maintain prolonged contact with the skin and produces an emollient effect. An advantage of a hydrocarbon ointment base is that it will retain moisture in the skin. Examples of hydrocarbon bases include White Petrolatum USP and White Ointment USP.

Absorption bases have the ability to absorb water and are often W/O emulsions. They have the ability to allow aqueous solutions to be incorporated into them and provide an emollient effect. Examples of absorption bases include Hydrophilic Petrolatum USP and Lanolin USP.

Water removable (water washable) base are O/W emulsions and are the most commonly used type of ointment base. These ointment bases are easily removed from the skin, can be diluted with water, and allow the absorption of discharges from the skin (Hydrophilic Ointment USP).

A water-soluble ointment base consists of soluble components or may include jelled aqueous solutions. These ointment bases are water washable and leave no water-insoluble residue. Polyethylene Glycol Ointment NF is an example of a water-soluble base.

169

An ointment is prepared by dispersing the drug uniformly throughout the vehicle base. The drug material is a fine powder or is present in a solution before it is incorporated into the vehicle base. The drug is incorporated into the ointment base through the process of levigation.

A cream is another topical dosage form that may be a viscous liquid or a semisolid emulsion (O/W or W/O). A pharmaceutical cream is classified by the USP as a water removable base. Often creams are used for cosmetic purposes. O/W creams are used as hand and foundation cream; W/O creams include cold and emollient creams.

Lab Activity #11.16: Compounding an ointment

Prepare 4 ounces of the following formula:

Salicylic acid		2%
White petrolatum	qs	4 ounces

Equipment needed:
- Calculator
- Disinfecting agent/cleanser
- Latex gloves
- Lint-free paper towels
- Metric weights
- Ointment jar
- Ointment slab or parchment paper
- Salicylic acid
- Spatula
- Sink with running hot and cold water
- Torsion or electronic balance
- Wedgwood mortar and pestle
- Weighing boats
- White petrolatum

Procedure
1. Perform the necessary calculations for the prescription.
2. Organize materials on workbench.
3. Wash hands and dry thoroughly.
4. Place gloves on hands.
5. Weigh proper quantity of salicylic acid in weighing boat on torsion or electronic balance.
6. Transfer salicylic acid to Wedgwood mortar and pestle, and triturate.
7. Weigh proper quantity of white petrolatum in a weighing boat on torsion or electronic balance.
8. Transfer white petrolatum to corner of ointment slab or parchment paper.
9. Add salicylic acid to other corner of ointment slab or parchment paper.
10. Add a small amount of the white petrolatum to the salicylic acid, and mix thoroughly using an "S" pattern with the spatula.
11. Continue adding white petrolatum to white petrolatum–salicylic acid compound, and mix thoroughly.
12. Ointment should not appear to have a gritty appearance; if it does, continue to mix it until the ointment has a uniform consistency.
13. Transfer ointment to an ointment jar of proper size. The top of the ointment in the ointment jar should be smooth and level.
14. Label the ointment jar.
15. Complete the compounding log.
16. Clean equipment and put away.

Time needed to complete this activity: 20 minutes

Pharmacy Compounding Log							
Drug Name	**Lot Number**	**Mfg. Expiration Date**	**Quantity Prepared**	**Measured by**	**Verified by**	**Beyond-Use Date**	

Compounding an Ointment Evaluation	Yes/No
Calculations correct	
Hands washed, dried, and gloved	
Correct quantity of salicylic acid weighed	
Salicylic acid triturated to a fine powder	
Correct quantity of white petrolatum weighed	
Salicylic acid and white petrolatum transferred to ointment slab or parchment paper	
Used "S" motion to incorporate salicylic acid into white petrolatum	
Texture of salicylic acid–white petrolatum compound is evenly mixed. No visible signs of salicylic acid powder. Ointment is not gritty.	
Salicylic acid–white petrolatum ointment transferred to ointment jar of proper size	
Final product has an eloquent appearance	
Ointment jar labeled properly	
Compounding log completed	
Equipment cleaned and put away	

12 Aseptic Technique

REINFORCE KEY CONCEPTS

TERMS AND DEFINITIONS

Select the correct term from the following list and write the corresponding letter in the blank next to the statement.

A. Aseptic technique
B. Clean room
C. Compounded sterile products
D. Gauge
E. Horizontal laminar flow hood
F. Hyperalimentation
G. Laminar flow hood
H. Nosocomial infection
I. Parenteral medication
J. Peripheral parenteral
K. Precipitate
L. Standard Precautions
M. Total parenteral nutrition
N. Vertical laminar flow hood

_D_ 1. The size of the needle opening

_G_ 2. Environment for preparation of sterile products within a streamline flow near a solid boundary

_F_ 3. Parenteral nutrition for individuals unable to eat

_L_ 4. A set of standards used in the preparation of medications that reduces the chance of contamination

_I_ 5. Medications administered by injection, such as intravenously or intramuscularly; introduced in a manner other than by way of the intestines

_A_ 6. The procedure used to eliminate the possibility of contamination of a drug with microbes or particles

_M_ 7. Large-volume IV nutrition administered through the central vein, which allows for higher concentrations of solutions

_E_ 8. Environment for preparation of sterile products that uses air originating from the back of the hood and moving forward across the hood out into the room

_J_ 9. Injection of a medication into the veins on the periphery of the body instead of into a central vein or artery

_N_ 10. Environment for preparation of chemotherapy treatments that uses air originating from the roof of the hood, moving downward and captured in a vent on the floor of the hood

_B_ 11. A contained and controlled environment within the pharmacy that has a low level of environmental pollutants

_K_ 12. To separate from solution or suspension

_C_ 13. Preparations prepared in a sterile environment using nonsterile ingredients or devices that must be sterilized before administration

_H_ 14. Infection that is obtained, after it has been admitted into an institution, by an unknown source

TRUE OR FALSE

Write T or F next to each statement.

___F___ 1. One of the most trivial responsibilities that a hospital pharmacy technician can have is the proper preparation of parenteral medications.

___F___ 2. All parenteral and ophthalmic medications should be prepared within a laminar flow hood.

___T___ 3. Cost can be a determining factor in the choice of some pharmacy equipment.

___T___ 4. All syringes must have a transfer needle if transported out of the pharmacy.

___F___ 5. Flexible bags and bottles are the main types of piggyback containers.

___F___ 6. Most syringes are made of glass and are meant to be sterilized and reused.

___T___ 7. The main purpose of needles in the pharmacy is to draw solution up into the syringe or to transfer solution from a syringe into a vial or other compatible container.

___F___ 8. To ensure sterility, the needle shaft must be wiped with alcohol.

___T___ 9. All chemotherapeutic agents should be prepared in a vertical flow hood.

___T___ 10. All IV rooms have references that can be used to find special instructions for all types of parenteral medications.

MULTIPLE CHOICE

Complete each question by circling the best answer.

1. An *MDV* is a:
   A. Multiple-drug vehicle
   B. Multiple-dose vial
   C. Metered dose ventilator
   D. None of the above

2. Which of the following is *not* a parenteral route of administration?
   A. IV
   B. IM
   C. SL
   D. SubQ

3. Nitroglycerin must be put only into:
   A. Glass containers
   B. Small-volume drips
   C. Syringe pumps
   D. Viaflex bags

4. Which of the following is *not* an example of a medication administration system?
   A. IV chamber
   B. CRIS
   C. CAD pump
   D. None of the above

5. A chunk of rubber from the vial stopper is dislodged and falls into the vial; this is called:
   A. Filtering
   B. Beveling
   C. Coring
   D. Piggybacking

6. To ensure sterility, which part of the needle should not be touched?
   A. Hub
   B. Shaft
   C. Bevel
   D. All of the above

7. When aseptic technique is used, what should not be worn?
   A. Gloves
   B. Artificial nails
   C. Hair ties
   D. All of the above

8. For proper hand washing technique, you should wash which areas for 30 to 90 seconds?
   A. Hands, face, and arms
   B. Hands, wrists, and arms
   C. Fingernails, wrists, and underarms
   D. Fingernails, hands, and face

9. To clean the hood, you should use:
   A. Soap and water
   B. Antimicrobial soap and hot water
   C. 70% isopropyl alcohol
   D. Hydrogen peroxide

10. The Julian date is:
    A. The actual consecutive day of the year
    B. Julian's birthday
    C. January 1
    D. December 31

FILL IN THE BLANK

Answer each question by completing the statement in the space provided.

1. All parenteral medications should be prepared in a manner that reduces the possibility of _____.

2. Large-volume drips include four sizes: _____, _____, _____, and _____.

3. Microdrip chambers are used most often for _____ patients.

4. A _____ dose of a patient-controlled analgesia (PCA) regimen is a preset amount of drug that can be administered by the patient when pain intensifies.

5. Two types of syringes that are commercially available are _____ and _____.

6. The rule to remember when sizing needles is that the gauge (size) number of the needle is _____ _____ to the needle's bore size.

7. The smallest filter is the _____ filter.

8. Aseptic technique goes hand-in-hand with _____ _____.

9. All work done in the hood is to be done _____ within the hood.

10. What type of filter is used in the hood to trap all particles larger than 0.2 μm? _____.

SHORT ANSWER

Write a short response to each question in the space provided.

1. Name two types of hyperalimentation: _____ and _____.

2. When preparing chemotherapy agents, you must wear _____ and _____.

3. Needles are made of _____ or _____.

4. The _____ route is the most dangerous to the patient because it bypasses the body's most

   _____ barriers and directly enters the _____.

5. A _____ _____ is used to draw up medications from an _____.

6. What is the process for breaking an ampule?

   _____

   _____

   _____

7. How are chemotherapy wastes disposed of?

   _____

   _____

   _____

8. Why are dextrose, amino acids, and lipids used in TPNs?

   _____

   _____

9. Why are syringes not reused when a change is made from one drug to another?

   _____

   _____

10. Why is the placement of the hands so important when sterile products are prepared?

   _____

   _____

RESEARCH ACTIVITY

Follow the instructions given in each exercise and provide a response.
Access the websites *www.usp797.org* and *www.globalrph.com/aseptic.htm*.

1. What is USP 797 all about?

2. Based on what you learned, describe aseptic technique.

3. List some precautions for patient care.

REFLECT CRITICALLY

CRITICAL THINKING

Reply to each question based on what you have learned in the chapter.

1. You have been preparing injections in the IV room and suddenly stick your finger with a needle. What went wrong? What mistake did you make that caused you to stick your finger?

   Lost focus, got distracted. Definitely were not practicing aseptic technique which would have prevented such accidents from occurring. Never try to attach needles in the air, always on the table.

2. If you stick your finger with a sterile needle, is it necessary to go to the emergency department for treatment?

   Yes you have to get your finger looked at for any risk of infection, even more so if you made yourself bleed.

3. You have been assigned to work in the IV preparation room for your shift. What are the first items you need to take care of when you walk into the IV room? What aseptic technique requirements need to be followed before you begin preparation of IVs?

   You must not be sick. You must wash your hands for 30-90 seconds. Clean the flow hood w/ 70% isopropyl alcohol. Make sure clothes are clean and more or less lint free. Check orders for the day and start making calculations based on stock.

177

4. What should you do at the end of your shift to ensure a smooth workflow when your replacement technician comes to relieve you? *Restock everything you used and clean everything as if you were never there. Leave no trace of your shift.*

LAB SCENARIOS

Pharmacy Equipment Used in Preparation of Sterile Compounds

Objective: To familiarize the pharmacy technician with equipment used in the preparation of sterile compounds.

Parenteral dosage forms differ from all other drug dosage forms because they are injected directly into body tissues through the skin and mucous membranes. Some of the many routes by which parenteral medications are injected into the body include intravenous, intramuscular, subcutaneous, and intradermal. Parenteral dosage forms differ from other pharmaceutical dosage forms for the following reasons:

- All products must be sterile.
- All products must be free from pyrogenic contamination.
- Injectable solutions must be free from visible particulate matter.
- Parenteral products should be isotonic; however, the degree of isotonicity will vary according to the route of administration of the medication.
- All parenteral products must be stable chemically, physically, and microbiologically.
- These products must be compatible with IV diluents, delivery systems, and other drug products that are coadministered.

Pharmacy technicians need to be familiar with various solutions that serve as vehicles for parenteral drugs. In addition, the technician must be familiar with equipment used in sterile compounding and its purpose.

Lab Activity #12.1: Identify the meaning of the following abbreviations used as infusion liquids.

Equipment needed:

- Pen/pencil

Time needed to complete this activity: 10 minutes

1. BWFI _____

2. SWFI _____

3. D5W _____

4. D10W _____

5. D20W _____

6. D5LR _____

7. D5 ¼ S _____

8. D5 ½ S _____

9. D5NS _____

10. D5R _____

11. D10NS _____

12. LR _____

13. R _____

14. NS _____

15. SOD Cl.5 _____

16. Sod Lac _____

Lab Activity #12.2: Correctly identify equipment used in the preparation of sterile compounds and its purpose.

Equipment needed:

- Administration set
- Alcohol pads
- Ampule
- Depth filter
- Disinfecting cleaning solution
- Filter needle
- Filter straw
- Gloves (powder free)
- Gown
- Hair cover
- Hypodermic needle
- Hypodermic syringe
- In-line filter
- Insulin syringe
- Intravenous piggyback
- Large-volume parenteral
- Mask
- Membrane filter
- Multiple-dose vial
- Nonsterile gauze swabs
- Nonvented administration set
- Port adapters
- Scrubs
- Sharps container
- Shoe covers
- Single dose vial
- Small-volume parenteral
- Sterile gauze swabs
- Syringe caps
- Transfer needle
- Tuberculin syringe
- Vented administration set

Time needed to complete this activity: 30 minutes

Equipment	Correctly Identified (Yes/No)	Purpose
Administration set		
Alcohol pads		
Ampule		
Depth filter		
Disinfecting cleaning solutions		
Filter needle		
Filter straw		
Gloves		
Gown		
Hair cover		
Hypodermic needle		

Equipment	Correctly Identified (Yes/No)	Purpose
Hypodermic syringe		
In-line filter		
Insulin syringe		
Intravenous piggyback		
Large-volume parenteral (LVP)		
Mask		
Membrane filter		
Multiple-dose vial		
Nonsterile gauze swabs		
Nonvented administration set		
Port adapters		
Scrubs		
Sharps container		
Shoe covers		
Single dose vial		
Small-volume parenteral (SVP)		
Sterile gauze swabs		
Syringe caps		
Transfer needle		
Tuberculin syringe		
Vented administration set		

Lab Activity #12.3: Correctly identify parts of a needle.

Equipment needed:

- Needle

Time needed to complete this activity: 5 minutes

Parts of a Needle	Correctly Identified (Yes/No)
Bevel	
Heel	
Hub	
Lumen	

Lab Activity #12.4: Correctly identify parts of a syringe.

Equipment needed:

- Tuberculin syringe

Time needed to complete this activity: 5 minutes

Parts of a Syringe	Correctly Identified (Yes/No)
Barrel	
Plunger	
Tip	

Proper Hand Washing in Aseptic Compounding

Objective: To perform a complete hand washing procedure as necessary before extemporaneous compounding.

The United States Pharmacopeia (USP) is a nongovernmental, official public standards-setting authority for prescription and over-the-counter medicines and other health care products manufactured in the United States. The USP establishes standards for the quality, purity, strength, and consistency of these products. The United States Pharmacopeia publishes the USP-NF, which is the official compendium for the United States. Chapter 797 of the USP addresses sterile compounding and is designed to cut down on infections transmitted to patients through pharmaceutical products. USP 797 addresses appropriate hand washing before preparation of compounded sterile products.

Lab Activity #12.5: Hand washing

Equipment needed:

- Biohazard waste container
- Disinfecting agent/cleanser
- Lint-free paper towels
- Nailbrush
- Sink with hot and cold running water

Procedure

1. Remove all jewelry, watches, and objects up to the elbow.
2. Turn on water faucets with a paper towel if not foot operated.
3. Make sure water temperature is lukewarm.
4. Avoid unnecessary splashing during washing process.
5. Apply sufficient disinfecting/cleansing agent to hands in a circular motion, holding the fingertips downward.
6. Clean all four surfaces of each finger, and rub well between the fingers.
7. Use a nailbrush to clean under every fingertip.
8. Clean all surfaces of hands, wrists, and arms up to the elbows in a circular motion.
9. Rinse well.
10. Repeat the scrubbing process a second time and rinse.
11. Dry hands with paper towels.
12. Do not touch the sink, faucet, or other objects that could contaminate hands.
13. Turn off water using a paper towel.
14. Discard paper towels in biohazard waste container.

Time needed to complete this activity: 10 minutes

Evaluation of Hand Washing	Yes/No
Removed all jewelry, watches, and objects up to the elbow	
Was not wearing acrylic nails or nail polish	
Started water and adjusted to the correct temperature	
Avoided unnecessary splashing during process	
Used sufficient disinfecting agent/cleanser	
Cleaned all four surfaces of each finger	
Cleaned all surfaces of hands, wrists, and arms up to the elbows in a circular motion	
Did not touch the sink, faucet, or other objects that could contaminate the hands	
Rinsed off all soap residue	
Rinsed hands, holding them upright and allowing water to drip to the elbow	
Did not turn off water until hands were completely dry	
Turned water off with a clean, dry, lint-free paper towel	
Did not touch the faucet while turning off the water	

Sterile Compounding

Objective: Demonstrate the proper sterile compounding techniques in performing a straight draw, reconstituting a powdered vial, and withdrawing a medication from an ampule.

Lab Activity #12.6: Performing a straight draw

Equipment needed:

- Alcohol swabs
- Biohazard container
- Disinfecting agent/cleanser
- Horizontal laminar airflow hood
- Isopropyl alcohol 70%
- Lint-free paper towels
- Personal protective equipment (foot covers, head cover, mask, gown, and sterile latex or latex-free gloves)
- Sharps container
- Single or multidose vial
- Sink with running hot and cold water
- Sterile gauze pad
- Sterile water
- Syringe with needle

Procedure

1. Gather all materials needed for manipulation.
2. Wash hands using proper technique.
3. Don PPEs.
4. Clean laminar airflow workbench.
5. Check the expiration of the single or multidose vial.
6. The next nine steps are conducted in the laminar airflow workbench area.
7. Swab the rubber top with alcohol. Allow the alcohol to dry.
8. Make sure the needle is firmly attached to the syringe.
9. Pull the plunger back on the syringe to slightly less than the amount needed to be drawn up.
10. Remove the needle cap. Find the center of the stopper and position the needle with the bevel end up.
11. Slightly bend the needle and insert the needle through the stopper.
12. Gently push the air from the syringe into the vial.
13. Pull back on the stopper until the desired amount is withdrawn.
14. Remove air bubbles.
15. Withdraw the needle and carefully recap.
16. Discard syringe in sharps container.
17. Remove PPEs in proper sequence.

Time needed to complete this activity: 20 minutes

Evaluation of a Straight Draw	Yes/No
Gather materials	
Wash hands	
Don PPEs	
Clean laminar airflow workbench	
Clean rubber top of vial with alcohol swab	
Select syringe of proper size	
Pull plunger back to slightly half of amount to be withdrawn	
Remove needle cap	
Insert needle into rubber stopper of vial	
Push air from plunger into vial	

Evaluation of a Straight Draw	Yes/No
Withdraw correct volume of medication	
Tap air bubbles out of syringe	
Withdraw needle and recap	
Discard syringe/needle in sharps container	

Lab Activity #12.7: Using a syringe and needle of proper size, remove the following volumes from a multidose vial within a laminar flow workbench.

Equipment needed:

- Alcohol swabs
- Horizontal laminar airflow workbench
- Multidose vial
- Syringes of multiple sizes with needle
- PPEs (foot covers, head cover, mask, gown, and sterile latex or latex-free gloves)
- Sharps container

Time needed to complete this activity: 10 minutes

Prescribed Volume	Measured Volume
0.25 ml	
0.5 ml	
0.75 ml	
1.2 ml	
1.5 ml	

Lab Activity #12.8: Reconstituting a powdered vial

Equipment needed:

- Alcohol swabs
- Laminar airflow hood
- PPEs (foot covers, head cover, mask, gown, and sterile latex or latex-free gloves)
- Sharps container
- Single or multidose vial
- Sink with running hot and cold water
- Syringe with needle
- Vented needle

Procedure

1. Gather all materials needed for manipulation.
2. Wash hands properly.
3. Don PPEs.
4. Check that laminar airflow workbench is cleaned properly.
5. Check the expiration date on the powdered vial and diluent.
6. Select syringe of proper size. (Note: The syringe should not exceed five times the volume of the drug to be withdrawn into the syringe.)
7. The next fifteen steps are to be completed within the laminar flow workbench.
8. Swab the rubber top with alcohol. Allow the alcohol to dry.
9. Make sure the needle is firmly attached to the syringe.
10. Prepare the syringe by adding the amount of air that will be equal to the amount of diluent to be withdrawn into the syringe.
11. Hold the syringe with the thumb and the index and middle fingers.
12. Remove cap from needle.
13. Insert the needle at a 45-degree angle into the rubber stopper of the vial with beveled part of the needle facing upward.
14. Hold the vial with the hand that is opposite the hand holding the syringe.

15. Push the plunger, forcing the air in the syringe into the vial, and release, gently allowing the fluid to be drawn into the syringe.
16. Tap the syringe to force air bubbles out of it.
17. Draw up the correct amount of diluent needed for reconstitution.
18. Pull back on the plunger to clear the neck of the syringe. Remove the needle and replace with a vented needle.
19. Remove all excess air from syringe.
20. Swab the top of the powdered vial with an alcohol swab.
21. Insert vented needle of the syringe at a 45-degree angle into the rubber top of the powdered vial.
22. Gently shake or swirl to dissolve. The powder must dissolve completely.
23. Place needle and syringe into the sharps container.
24. Remove PPEs in proper order, and discard appropriately.

Time needed to complete this activity: 20 minutes

Evaluation of Reconstituting a Powdered Vial	Yes/No
Materials gathered properly	
Hands washed	
PPEs donned properly	
Laminar airflow workbench cleaned	
Checked expiration dates of medications	
Vial top cleaned	
Correct needles used during reconstitution	
Air bubbles removed from syringe	
Correct amount and type of diluent added to vial per directions on the vial	
Powder dissolved	
Syringe and needle disposed into sharps container	

Lab Activity #12.9: Ampule preparation

Equipment needed:

- Alcohol swabs
- Ampule
- Filter needle
- Laminar airflow hood
- PPEs (foot covers, head cover, mask, gown, and sterile latex or latex-free gloves)
- Sharps container
- Sink with running hot and cold water
- Syringe with needle

Procedure
1. Gather all materials needed for activity.
2. Wash hands properly.
3. Don PPEs in the proper sequence.
4. Clean laminar flow workbench in the proper manner using the correct supplies and techniques.
5. Check the expiration date of the ampule.
6. Tap the top of the ampule, forcing all liquid at the top and neck of the ampule to fall into the body of the ampule.
7. Clean the neck of the ampule with an alcohol swab.
8. Hold the body of the ampule with your thumb and index finger.
9. Using your stronger hand, place the thumb and forefinger over the top of the ampule.
10. Apply pressure to the neck of the ampule with a sudden motion of the wrist.
11. Place the head of the ampule into the sharps container, and place the ampule on the work surface of the laminar flow workbench.
12. Hold the barrel of the syringe with the hand and remove the cap of the needle.
13. Place cap onto the alcohol swab with the opening pointing toward the HEPA filter of the hood.

14. Hold barrel of syringe so the needle is pointing downward.
15. Cautiously insert the needle into the ampule so the needle is entered into the fluid of the ampule.
16. Pull the plunger of the syringe until the syringe contains more than the desired volume.
17. Hold ampule with your other hand as the first hand holds the barrel of the syringe and releases the plunger.
18. Remove the syringe from the ampule, invert the syringe upward, and recap.
19. Remove air bubbles from the syringe by tapping it.
20. Pull plunger downward, causing fluid from the ampule to enter into the syringe.
21. Push remaining air from the syringe by releasing the plunger.
22. Attach a filter needle to the syringe.
23. Remove excess air and cap syringe.
24. Clean port of IV bag with alcohol swab.
25. Inject drug into IV bag.
26. Discard syringe into sharps container.
27. Remove PPEs in the proper sequence, and discard.

Time needed to complete this activity: 20 minutes

Evaluation of Ampule Preparation	Yes/No
Followed proper hand washing procedures and techniques	
Wore appropriate PPEs	
Followed proper procedure and technique in cleaning the hood	
Performed all necessary calculations correctly prior to drug preparation	
Brought the correct drugs and concentrations into the hood for preparation	
Checked expiration dates of medications	
Brought the correct supplies into the hood prior to preparation	
Inspected all products for particulate matter/contamination prior to use	
Cleaned ampule neck correctly before breaking	
Wrapped ampule neck correctly before breaking	
Broke ampule correctly	
Attached filter device to syringe correctly	
Drew up ampule correctly without spilling contents	
Removed filter needle and replaced it with new needle before injecting final container	
Drew up correct amount of drug and checked measurement before injecting into container	
Cleaned additive port on final container before injecting drug	
Did not core or puncture side of additive port when adding drug to the final container	
Properly mixed contents of container and inspected for incompatibilities or particulate matter	
Properly sealed additive port of container	
Did not contaminate the needle or syringe during preparation	
Did not contaminate the laminar airflow hood	
Did not at any time block airflow from HEPA filter or air intake grills	
Did not utilize the outer 6 inches of the hood opening	
Properly discarded waste, including sharps	
Removed PPEs in proper sequence	
Discarded PPEs in appropriate container	

Chapter **12** **Aseptic Technique**

Personal Protective Equipment (PPEs)

Objective: Identify personal protective equipment, explain its purpose in sterile compounding, and demonstrate proper techniques in donning personal protective equipment in the correct sequence.

The Occupational Safety and Health Administration requires the use of personal protective equipment (PPE) to reduce the exposure of employees to hazards. In the practice of pharmacy, PPEs are worn in the compounding of sterile products. These PPEs include foot and hair covers, face masks, gowns, and latex (latex-free) gloves.

Gowns are worn to protect the skin and to prevent soiling of clothing during procedures that are likely to generate splashes. Masks, eye protection, and face shields are worn to protect the mucous membranes of the eyes, nose, and mouth during procedures that are likely to produce splashes. In addition, masks prevent moisture from being forced out from the mouth and nose during normal activities such as breathing or talking. Gloves are worn to prevent the spread of disease and to avoid possible contamination. However, the individual who wears gloves must still wash his/her hands before gloving. A pharmacy technician should never wash his/her hands with gloves on, because hand washing may damage the glove's pores, allowing microorganisms to enter the glove.

Lab Activity #12.10: Identify the following personal protective equipment worn in the practice of sterile compounding, and state its purpose.

Equipment needed:

- Face mask
- Foot coverings
- Goggles
- Hair covering
- Sterile gown
- Sterile latex or latex-free gloves

Time needed to complete this activity: 5 minutes

Personal Protective Equipment	Purpose
Face mask	
Foot coverings	
Goggles	
Hair covering	
Sterile gown	
Sterile latex (latex-free) gloves	

Lab Activity #12.11: Donning personal protective equipment

Equipment needed:

- Disinfecting agent/cleanser
- Face mask
- Foam alcohol
- Foot covering
- Hair covering
- Lint-free paper towels
- Nailbrush
- Sink with hot and cold running water
- Sterile gown
- Sterile latex (or latex-free) gloves

Procedure

1. Remove all jewelry up to the elbows and remove necklaces and earrings; earrings should not be larger than a quarter in diameter.
2. Remove all outer garments such as coats and hats.
3. Wash hands thoroughly with soap and water.
4. Pull shoe cover over the toe of the shoe first, around the bottom of the shoe, and finally over the heel of the shoe. Please note that shoe covers are not designated as left and right but are interchangeable.
5. Put on hair cover by gathering loose hair and placing it into the back of the hair cover. Pull front of hair cover over forehead. No hair should be outside of the hair cover.
6. Slip on face mask by situating the top of the mask at the bridge of the nose. Pull the two top ties of the face mask and attach them together. Attach the two lower ties behind the neck. The mask should cover the nose, mouth, and chin.
7. Wash hands using the techniques performed in lab number 12.5.
8. Open the package of the sterile gown. The gown should never make contact with any surface.
9. Slip one arm into the sleeve of the sterile gown, and pull it up to the shoulder. Repeat this procedure with the other arm. Tie the neck strings behind the neck, and repeat with the waist strings.
10. Apply foam alcohol to the palm of one hand, and rub hands thoroughly. Allow hands to air dry.
11. Open package containing sterile latex (or latex-free) gloves. Remove glove from package and maintain fingers within the cup of the gown. Place glove on palm of hand with the thumb side of the glove toward the palm. Pull the glove's cuff so that it covers the gown's cuff. Unfold the glove's cuff so that it covers the cuff of the gown. Take hold of the glove and gown at waist level. Pull glove onto the hand and work fingers into the glove. Repeat procedure for the other glove.

Time needed to complete this activity: 15 minutes

Evaluation of Donning Personal Protective Equipment	Yes/No
Jewelry removed	
Hands washed properly	
Shoe covers put on	
Hair cover put on properly	
Face mask put on properly	
Aseptic hand washing performed	
Sterile gown put on properly	
Foam alcohol applied	
Sterile gloves put on properly	

Lab Activity #12.12: Removal of personal protective equipment

Equipment needed:

- Hair covering
- Sterile gown
- Sterile latex (or latex-free) gloves
- Face mask
- Foot covering
- Biohazard container

Procedure

1. Use your dominant hand to grasp the glove of the opposite hand near the palm.
2. Pull glove inside out until you reach your fingers.
3. Place your thumb of the nongloved hand inside the cuff of the other glove. Pull glove inside out until you reach your fingers and pull over the first removed glove.
4. Dispose of gloves in biohazard container.
5. Remove gown.

Chapter **12** **Aseptic Technique**

6. Remove face mask.
7. Remove hair cover.
8. Remove shoe covers
9. Dispose of gown, face mask, hair cover, and shoe covers in biohazard container.

Time needed to complete this activity: 5 minutes

Evaluation of Personal Protective Equipment Removal	Yes/No
Glove removed and disposed of properly	
Gown removed correctly	
Face mask removed properly	
Hair cover removed correctly	
Shoe covers removed properly	
Personal protective equipment disposed of appropriately	

Laminar Airflow Workbench

Objective: Demonstrate the proper cleaning of a horizontal laminar airflow workbench.

A laminar airflow workbench is used in the compounding of sterile products. Laminar airflow workbenches are used to filter bacteria and other particulate matter from the air and to maintain constant airflow out of the hood to prevent contamination. Several types of laminar airflow workbenches are available, including vertical (biological safety cabinet) and horizontal laminar airflow cabinets. Both types of flow hoods are built to allow the flow of sterile air across a work surface. Air particles are removed through the use of a high-efficiency particulate air (HEPA) filter. HEPA filters should be tested every 6 months.

The vertical or biological safety cabinet (BSC) is used in the preparation of chemotherapeutic agents and antineoplastic agents. The vertical airflow workbench filters air from the top down to the workbench and can remove particles 0.3 microns and larger. Horizontal laminar flow workbenches are the most common type used in the preparation of sterile products; they are capable of filtering particulate matter of 0.2 microns or larger. They blow air from the back of the hood to the front of the hood. Horizontal laminar flow workbenches are less likely to wash organisms into the sterility test media. Unfortunately, any airborne particulate matter generated in the unit is blown into both the pharmacy personnel and the room. Regardless of the type of laminar flow workbench used, the pharmacist or pharmacy technician must be trained properly on its uses and proper maintenance. A laminar airflow workbench must be turned on for at least 30 minutes before it is used.

Lab Activity #12.13: Cleaning a horizontal laminar airflow hood

Equipment needed:

- Disinfecting agent/cleanser
- Horizontal laminar airflow hood
- Isopropyl alcohol 70%
- Lint-free paper towels
- PPEs (foot covers, head cover, mask, gown, and sterile latex or latex-free gloves)
- Sink with running hot and cold water
- Sterile water
- Sterile gauze pad

Procedure

1. Turn horizontal laminar airflow workbench on for at least 30 minutes.
2. Wash hands using techniques demonstrated in lab 12.5.
3. Deposit sterile, lint-free cleaning pads 6 inches inside laminar workflow.
4. Moisten lightly sterile gauze pads with sterile water.
5. Take moist gauze pads and begin to clean the back inside corner of laminar workbench, beginning with the ceiling. Cleaning should be performed using overlapping side-to-side motions. After ceiling has been cleaned, discard gauze pads.

6. Use moist gauze pads to clean the right-side section with overlapping up-down motion beginning in the back corner, and move forward to front of laminar airflow workbench; discard used gauze pads.
7. Repeat process on the left-side section of laminar airflow workbench, beginning in the back corner, with overlapping up-down motion; move forward. Discard dirty gauze pads.
8. Repeat process on the work surface of the workbench. Begin in the back right-hand corner, going side-to-side with overlapping motion. Clean to the outer edge of the laminar airflow workbench.
9. Repeat steps 5 through 8 in the same order, using 70% isopropyl alcohol instead of sterile water.
10. Record initials, date, and time on the cleaning log.

Time needed to complete this activity: 20 minutes

Cleaning Log		
Date of Laminar Airflow Cleaning	**Time of Cleaning**	**Initials of Person Completing the Cleaning**

Evaluation of Cleaning a Horizontal Laminar Airflow Hood	Yes/No
Hood turned on and running at least 30 minutes prior to preparation	
Proper hand washing procedure followed	
Personal protective equipment donned in proper sequence and worn	
Clean, sterile gauze/sponge and disinfectant used to clean the hood	
Clean ceiling using sterile water and proper techniques	
Clean the right side of the hood using sterile water with the appropriate motions. Start at the top and work from side to side with overlapping strokes.	
Clean left side of hood using sterile water with correct motions. Start at the top and work from side to side with overlapping strokes.	
Clean the work surface last using sterile water and appropriate strokes. Start at the back and work from side to side with overlapping strokes.	
Clean ceiling with 70% isopropyl alcohol and proper technique.	
Clean right side with 70% isopropyl alcohol with appropriate motions. Start at the top and work from side to side with overlapping strokes.	
Clean left side of hood using 70% isopropyl alcohol with correct motions. Start at the top and work from side to side with overlapping strokes.	
Clean the work surface last using 70% isopropyl alcohol and water with appropriate strokes. Start at the back and work from side to side with overlapping strokes.	
Were previously cleaned surfaces contaminated?	
Was the airflow from HEPA filter blocked?	
Complete cleaning log.	

Chapter **12** Aseptic Technique

1. What is the difference between a vertical and a horizontal laminar airflow hood? When should they be used?

_____

_____

_____

_____

_____

_____

2. In what direction does air flow in a horizontal airflow workbench?

_____

3. In what direction does air flow in a vertical airflow workbench?

_____

4. How often should the HEPA filter be checked?

_____

Preparing Small- and Large-Volume Parenterals

Objective: To introduce the pharmacy technician to the preparation of small- and large-volume parenterals.

> The most common type of sterile product prepared by a pharmacy technicians is an intravenous (IV) bag that contains a medication. Intravenous bags are classified as small volume or large volume. A small-volume IV bag contains a volume less than 100 milliliters; a large-volume IV bag contains 100 milliliters or more of a fluid. Some of the medications found in IV bags include antibiotics, antiviral agents, antineoplastics, and analgesics. During the preparation of IV bags, it is extremely important that aseptic techniques are followed.

Lab Activity #12.14: Prepare an intravenous compound.

Equipment needed:

- Alcohol swabs
- Diluent
- Filter needle
- Laminar airflow hood
- Large-volume parenteral (LVP) or small-volume parenteral (SVP)
- PPEs
- Sharps container
- Single dose vial (SDV) or multidose vial
- Sink with running hot and cold water
- Syringe with needle
- Vented needle

Procedure

1. Gather all materials needed for activity.
2. Wash hands properly.
3. Don PPEs in the proper sequence.
4. Clean laminar flow workbench in the proper manner, using the correct supplies and techniques.
5. Collect the medication to be compounded.
6. Check expiration dates on both the vial and the parenteral IV bag.
7. Place ingredients in the laminar flow hood.

   If you are right-handed, place them in the following order (going left to right):
   Diluent, single dose or multidose vial, alcohol swabs, syringe, IV bag

or

If you are left-handed, place them in the following order (going right to left):
Diluent, single dose or multidose vial, alcohol swabs, syringe, IV bag

8. Swab the rubber top with alcohol. Allow the alcohol to dry.
9. Make sure the needle is firmly attached to the syringe.
10. Prepare the syringe by adding the amount of air that will be equal to the amount of diluent to be withdrawn into the syringe.
11. Hold the syringe with the thumb and the index and middle fingers.
12. Remove cap from needle.
13. Insert the needle at a 45-degree angle into the rubber stopper of the vial with beveled part of the needle facing upward.
14. Hold the vial with the hand opposite the hand that is holding the syringe.
15. Invert the vial and pull back on the plunger.
16. Push the plunger, forcing the air in the syringe into the vial, and release gently, allowing the fluid to be drawn into the syringe.
17. Tap the syringe to force air bubbles out of it.
18. Draw up the correct amount of diluent needed for the reconstitution.
19. Transfer the diluent into the vial containing the medication.
20. Pull back on the plunger to clear the neck of the syringe. Remove the needle, and replace with a vented needle.
21. Remove all excess air from syringe.
22. Insert vented needle of the syringe at a 45-degree angle into the rubber top of the powdered vial.
23. Gently shake or swirl to dissolve. The powder must dissolve completely.
24. Draw into the syringe a volume of air that will displace the volume of medication being removed.
25. Clean the medication port of the IV bag with alcohol swab.
26. Inject medication into the medication port of the IV bag.
27. Discard syringe into sharps container.
28. Remove PPEs in the proper sequence, and discard.
29. Record initials, date, and time on the cleaning log.

Time needed to complete this activity: 20 minutes

Cleaning Log		
Date of Laminar Airflow Cleaning	**Time of Cleaning**	**Initials of Person Completing the Cleaning**

Evaluation of Intravenous Bag Preparation	**Yes/No**
Followed proper hand washing procedures and techniques	
Wore appropriate PPEs	
Followed proper procedure and technique in cleaning the hood	
Performed all necessary calculations correctly prior to drug preparation	
Brought the correct drugs and concentrations into the hood for preparation	
Checked expiration dates of medications	
Brought the correct supplies into the hood prior to preparation	
Inspected all products for particulate matter/contamination prior to use	
Removed filter needle and replaced it with new needle before injecting final container	
Drew up correct amount of drug and checked measurement before injecting into container	

Chapter **12** Aseptic Technique

Evaluation of Intravenous Bag Preparation	Yes/No
Cleaned additive port on final container before injecting drug	
Did not core or puncture side of additive port when adding drug to the final container	
Properly mixed contents of container and inspected for incompatibilities or particulate matter	
Properly sealed additive port of container	
Did not contaminate the needle or syringe during preparation	
Did not contaminate the laminar airflow hood	
Did not at any time block airflow from HEPA filter or air intake grills	
Did not utilize the outer 6 inches of the hood opening	
Properly discarded waste, including sharps	
Removed PPEs in proper sequence	
Discarded PPEs in appropriate container	
Completed cleaning log	

Preparing Cytotoxic Parenterals

Objective: To introduce the pharmacy technician to proper techniques in compounding cytotoxic parenteral medications and disposing of hazardous waste.

A pharmacy technician may be required to prepare an antineoplastic or cytotoxic medication for a patient diagnosed with a form of cancer. These agents are used to kill a specific type or form of cancer cell found in a patient. Although these agents have many benefits for the patient, they are unable to distinguish a cancer cell from a healthy cell. Therefore special measures must be taken to protect the pharmacist or pharmacy technician from being exposed to these agents accidentally.

Compounding cytotoxic medications is very similar to compounding sterile medications, with a few exceptions. First, cytotoxic compounds are prepared in biological safety cabinets (vertical laminar airflow workbench), which are similar to horizontal laminar airflow workbenches, with the primary exception being that the air is blown from the top of the hood vertically, which prevents fumes inside the hood. Biological safety cabinets (BSCs) may take the form of a glove box isolator, with which the pharmacist or pharmacy technician slips his/her hands into a glove-like component contained in the cabinet.

Many of the policies and procedures used in preparing a sterile compound are applied when cytotoxic agents are prepared.

Lab Activity #12.15: Cleaning a biological safety cabinet (BSC)

Equipment needed:

- 70% isopropyl alcohol
- Biological safety cabinet (a laminar airflow workbench in the absence of a biological safety cabinet)
- Biological safety cabinet cleaner
- Deionized water
- Germicidal cleanser
- Goggles
- Lint-free cloth
- Personal protective equipment
- Sink with running hot and cold water

Procedure

1. Gather all materials needed for activity.
2. Wash hands properly.
3. Don PPEs in the proper sequence.
4. **MAKE SURE THE BLOWER IS ON!**
5. Using the lint-free cloth, begin cleaning the bar at the top of the hood.

192

6. Move to the back panel of the hood, and clean the top of the panel in a side-to-side motion, moving toward the bottom.
7. Clean each side panel next, going from the top of the panel to the bottom of the panel.
8. Clean the base of the workbench, moving from the rear forward using a sideward motion.
9. Scrub from top to bottom of the workbench, using the cleaner.
10. Rinse cabinet with deionized water.
11. Repeat process with 70% isopropyl alcohol.
12. Record initials, date, and time on the cleaning log.

Time needed to complete this activity: 15 minutes

Cleaning Log		
Date of Laminar Airflow Cleaning	**Time of Cleaning**	**Initials of Person Completing the Cleaning**

Cleaning a Biological Safety Cabinet	Yes/No
Hands washed properly	
PPEs and goggles worn	
Biological safety cabinet blower on	
Lint-free cloth used	
Inside of biological safety cabinet cleaned in proper sequence	
Biological safety cabinet cleaner used inside of cabinet	
Biological cabinet is rinsed inside with deionized water	
70% isopropyl alcohol used to clean inside of biological safety cabinet	
Completed the cleaning log	

If a laminar airflow work bench is used, remember that in a hospital pharmacy, cytotoxic compounds are prepared in a biological safety cabinet.

Lab Activity #12.16: Vial preparation—hazardous drugs

Equipment needed:

- 70% isopropyl alcohol
- Biohazardous waste bag
- Biological safety cabinet (a laminar airflow workbench in the absence of a biological safety cabinet)
- Biological safety cabinet cleaner
- Calculator
- Chemo mat
- Chemo spill kit
- Deionized water
- Eyewash station
- Foil
- Gauze
- Germicidal cleanser
- Goggles
- Hazardous waste container
- Large-volume or small-volume parenteral IV bag
- Luer-Lok syringe with needle
- Lint-free cloth

Chapter **12** **Aseptic Technique**

- Personal protective equipment
- Sharps container
- Sink with running hot and cold water
- Vial
- Zip-Loc bag

Procedure

1. Gather all materials needed for activity.
2. All compounding calculations should be performed and checked by instructor.
3. Wash hands properly.
4. Don PPEs in the proper sequence.
5. Clean biological safety cabinet.
6. Place chemo mat inside of biological safety cabinet.
7. Check all ingredients for particulate matter and possible contamination.
8. Clean the top of the vial with alcohol swab.
9. Pull the plunger of the Luer-Lok syringe halfway back for the amount of drug to be drawn into the syringe.
10. Take off the cap from the needle.
11. Insert the needle into the center of the vial with the beveled tip of the needle up.
12. Hold vial so that air is being blown onto the syringe and the stopper of the vial.
13. Holding the syringe from the bottom, gradually push the air from the syringe into the vial.
14. Withdraw the correct amount of medication from the vial by slowly pulling the syringe's plunger back.
15. Remove the needle from the vial once the correct amount of drug has been measured.
16. Remove air bubbles from syringe.
17. Recap the syringe.
18. Clean medication port with alcohol swab.
19. Inject medication into IV bag.
20. Mix thoroughly the medication that has been injected into the IV bag.
21. Check for any particulate matter.
22. Clean the outside of the IV bag with moist gauze, as well as all IV ports.
23. Place a small piece of foil around the medication port.
24. Label final product, and place inside Zip-Loc bag.
25. Place used syringe and needle into sharps container.
26. Remove PPEs in proper sequence, and place in a hazardous waste container.
27. Record initials, date, and time on the cleaning log.

Time needed to complete this activity: 20 minutes

Cleaning Log		
Date of Laminar Airflow Cleaning	**Time of Cleaning**	**Initials of Person Completing the Cleaning**

Evaluation of Preparing a Hazardous Drug from a Vial	**Yes/No**
Eyewash station in compounding area	
Chemo spill kit in compounding area	
Compounding calculations checked by instructor	
Adhered to hand washing procedure	
PPEs and goggles worn	
Biological safety cabinet cleaned properly using correct tools and in proper sequence	
Chemo mat in biological safety cabinet	
Checked for possible contamination in vial and IV bag	

Evaluation of Preparing a Hazardous Drug from a Vial	Yes/No
Rubber diaphragm cleaned	
Needle inserted into vial properly to prevent possible coring	
Used a venting device that had a 0.2 micron hydrophobic filter	
Correct volume of medication drawn into syringe	
Air bubbles removed from syringe before removal of the syringe from the vial	
Needle removed from syringe, resulting in no spillage	
Medication port of IV bag cleaned before injecting medication into IV bag	
IV bag mixed thoroughly with no visible signs of particulate matter	
Final product labeled and placed in Zip-Loc bag	
Placed syringe in sharps container	
Removed PPEs and goggles in proper sequence	
Discarded PPEs in hazardous waste container	
Completed the cleaning log	

13 Pharmacy Stock and Billing

REINFORCE KEY CONCEPTS

TERMS AND DEFINITIONS

Select the correct term from the following list and write the corresponding letter in the blank next to the statement.

A. Adjudication
B. Formulary
C. Treatment authorization request
D. POS
E. Copay
F. Closed formulary
G. Drug utilization evaluation
H. National provider identifier
I. Pharmacy and Therapeutics Committee
J. Medicare Modernization Act
K. Prior authorization
L. Open formulary
M. Patient profile
N. Periodic automatic replenishment
O. Material safety data sheets

___C___ 1. The process/form used for Medicare and Medicaid to preapprove a drug, treatment, or therapy

___E___ 2. The portion of the prescription bill that the patient is responsible for paying

___A___ 3. Electronic insurance billing for medication payment

___D___ 4. Point of sale

___F___ 5. Medication use is tightly restricted to those medications provided within the formulary list

___B___ 6. A list of approved drugs to be stocked by the pharmacy; also, a list of drugs covered by an insurance company

___H___ 7. Number assigned to any health care provider; used for the purpose of standardizing health data transmissions

___M___ 8. List of necessary patient personal and health information

___L___ 9. Medication use is essentially unrestricted in the types of drug choices offered or prescribed

___G___ 10. Process by which pharmacist ensures proper medication utilization

___J___ 11. Enactment of prescription drug coverage to be paid out for persons covered under Medicare

___I___ 12. Medical staff composed of physicians and pharmacists who provide necessary information and advice on whether a drug should be added to a formulary

___K___ 13. Insurance-required approval for a restricted, non-formulary, or noncovered medication prior to time of filling

___N___ 14. Stock levels to a certain number of allowed units

___O___ 15. Information sheets supplied to the pharmacy from the manufacturer of chemical products, listing hazards and handling if exposed

TRUE OR FALSE

Write T or F next to each statement.

__T__ 1. A pharmacy technician often is put in charge of billing.

__F__ 2. A formulary is a book that contains compounding recipes.

__F__ 3. Most formulary drugs are generic drugs.

__F__ 4. Generic drugs are less expensive because they are less effective than brand name drugs.

__F__ 5. In a PPO, the patient must select a physician from the insurance plan's list.

__T__ 6. A PPO plan usually has a higher copayment than an HMO.

__F__ 7. If an insurance claim is rejected, the technician must call the help desk to find out why.

__T__ 8. Each insurance plan has specific guidelines that must be followed for reimbursement to be made.

__F__ 9. The cost of prescriptions is the same from pharmacy to pharmacy.

__T__ 10. A patient may call for a refill after 1 week from the day the person filled the prescription, as long as there are refills remaining.

__F__ 11. If the cardholder's information does not match up to the processor's information, the patient does not have coverage.

__T__ 12. Automated dispensing systems are switching over from entering personal identifying codes to using fingerprint ID.

__T__ 13. One of the best ways to learn drug names and to become familiar with the drugs' locations in your pharmacy is to put away new stock.

__F__ 14. Recall notices arrive by voice mail.

__T__ 15. Cytotoxic drugs require special packaging when they are returned to the manufacturer.

MULTIPLE CHOICE

Complete the question by circling the best answer.

1. Who is responsible for maintaining the inventory stock in the pharmacy?
   A. Pharmacist
   B. Technician
   C. Inventory technician
   D. All of the above

2. The types of drugs typically included in a formulary are:
   A. New drugs
   B. Generic drugs and common branded drugs for which no generic is available in the drug class
   C. Uncommon drugs
   D. Extremely expensive drugs

3. In third-party billing, the third party is the:
   A. Pharmacy
   B. Patient
   C. Insurance company
   D. All of the above

4. Which of the following is *not* a type of health insurance plan in use today?
   A. POS
   B. HMO
   C. PPO
   D. Medicare

5. Which of the following is *not* a special feature of an HMO?
   A. Primary care physician
   B. Independent physicians' association
   C. Copayment
   D. Workers' compensation

6. Which of the following is *not* a difference between HMOs and PPOs?
   A. A PPO plan has no requirements for a PCP
   B. PPO plans have a copayment
   C. PPO plans have a deductible
   D. All of the above

7. The amount a patient must pay before the copay starts is called the:
   A. Share of cost
   B. Penalty period
   C. Deductible
   D. Grace period

8. Which of the following is *not* a government-run insurance program?
   A. Medicare
   B. Medicaid
   C. Long-term disability
   D. Workers' compensation

9. Which group is *not* covered by Medicare?
   A. Healthy infants
   B. Disabled patients
   C. Seniors
   D. Dialysis patients

10. The insurance company decides the amount of coverage per medication based on:
   A. AWP
   B. Copay
   C. DAW
   D. A and B

11. Which of the following is *not* a reason for the insurance company to reject a claim?
   A. Coverage has expired
   B. Use of a generic drug
   C. Refill too soon
   D. NDC not covered

12. Some patients are exempt from insurance limitations because of their illness or disease. Which group of patients is *not* exempt?
    A. Diabetic patients
    B. Cancer patients
    C. HIV patients
    D. AIDS patients

13. Sometimes insurance companies refill medications early because:
    A. The patient lost the medication
    B. The patient is going on a vacation
    C. The physician told the patient to increase the dosage
    D. All of the above

14. Which of the following is *not* an example of an inventory system that can keep a running inventory of medications, as well as order them?
    A. SOC system
    B. POS system
    C. Order card system
    D. Handheld computer inventory system

15. Which of the following is *not* a reason to return medications to the warehouse or manufacturer?
    A. Drug recalled
    B. Drug damaged during delivery
    C. Drug incorrectly reconstituted
    D. Drug expired

16. Manufacturers are required by law to recall any product that has been found to have which of the following guideline violations?
    A. Labeling is wrong
    B. Product was not packaged or produced properly
    C. Drug batch was contaminated
    D. All of the above

17. Drug utilization evaluation (DUE) is an important process used to screen the medication order for:
    A. Duplicate therapy
    B. Possible errors
    C. Drug-drug interactions
    D. All of the above

18. A zero for a DAW code means:
    A. No refills
    B. Dispense order as written
    C. Generic substitution authorized
    D. Dispense brand name only

19. Point-of-sale billing allows the insurance company to:
    A. Price a claim
    B. Verify eligibility
    C. Identify covered drugs
    D. All of the above

20. Reasons for obtaining a prior authorization may include:
    A. Patient is demanding the drug
    B. Drug of choice not formulary
    C. Physician is requesting
    D. None of the above

FILL IN THE BLANK

Answer each question by completing the statement in the space provided.

1. An HMO is an effective method of controlling _____ _____ _____.

2. An HMO may require _____ authorization (PA) on certain medications.

3. The difference between HMOs and PPOs is that the patient usually pays more _____ _____ _____ for PPOs.

4. Each state has its own _____ program for low-income residents.

5. The information that insurance companies must have to process a claim from the pharmacy or to reimburse a patient is the same as on a _____ _____.

6. _____ _____ is a type of insurance paid by _____ to fully cover injuries suffered by _____ while on the job.

SHORT ANSWER

Write a short response to each question in the space provided.

1. When an insurance company is billing for medication, what is the minimum information the insurance company requires?_____

2. One of the most common problems resulting in a claim rejection is a non-ID match. What patient information should be double-checked in these cases? _____

3. Why do many pharmacies have a policy of pulling off the shelves any medication that will expire in 3 months or sooner? _____

4. What are the three main responsibilities of automated return companies?

A. _____

B. _____

C. _____

5. To what categories of drugs must the pharmacy give special consideration? Why?

_____

_____

6. What are the three Medicare levels available?

A. Medicare Part A

_____

B. Medicare Part B

_____

C. Medicare Part D

_____

7. What are the two types of Medicare Part D plans, as outlined by *Consumer Reports?*

_____

_____

_____

RESEARCH ACTIVITY

Follow the instructions given in each exercise and provide a response.

1. Access the website *www.fda.gov* for FDA news, recalls, and product safety.

A. Find and list three drugs that have been recalled.

B. What were the reasons for the recalls?

2. Make a phone call or speak to someone who has an HMO, PPO health insurance policy.

A. What is the drug coverage?

B. Is there a copay for generic/brand drugs?

REFLECT CRITICALLY

CRITICAL THINKING

Reply to each question based on what you have learned in the chapter.

1. Should Medicare cover all medical and prescription costs for elderly patients? Give three pros and three cons for this issue.

   1-P- elderly can live much more relaxed, healthy lives
   2-P- they can give more back to community/productivity
   3-P- can spend their money on other things to keep economy stable

   1-C- way too expensive
   2-C- unreasonable to do so, some may need very expensive drugs
   3-C- Elderly will feel inappropriate sense of entitlement and make unreasonable demands/requests (probably)

2. Many Canadian pharmacies are offering prescription drugs at vastly reduced prices compared with U.S. prices. Is there any reason not to "go across the border" for your medications?

   They may have different regulations regarding when a drug is deemed safe for public and put on the market. It may be risky and unsafe even though it's on the market, hence cheaper.

3. Choosing an insurance health plan can be overwhelming. What type of coverage would best meet your needs? Outline all items you would need to have total health coverage.

   Cheapest coverage that raes basically only emergencies. I am a healthy adult and am on no medication. I want the cheapest possible coverage for me and my insurance company.

LAB SCENARIOS

Purchase of Pharmaceuticals

Objective: To follow the legal requirements of ordering and receiving Schedule II medications and to become familiar with various types of medication recalls.

Lab Activity #13.1: Completion of a DEA Form 222

Equipment needed:

- Sample DEA Form 222
- *Physicians' Desk Reference* or *Drug Facts and Comparisons*
- Black ink pen

See Reverse of PURCHASER'S Copy for Instructions		No order form may be issued for Schedule I and II substances unless a completed application form has been received. (21 CFR 1305.04).		OMB APPROVAL No. 1117-0010
TO: *(Name of Supplier)*			STREET ADDRESS	
CITY and STATE		DATE	TO BE FILLED IN BY SUPPLIER	
			SUPPLIERS DEA REGISTRATION No.	

LINE No.	No. of Packages	Size of Package	Name of Item	National Drug Code	Packages Shipped	Date Shipped
			TO BE FILLED IN BY PURCHASER			
1						
2						
3						
4						
5						
6						
7						
8						
9						
10						

◄ LAST LINE COMPLETED *(MUST BE 10 OR LESS)* | SIGNATURE OF PURCHASER OR ATTORNEY OR AGENT

Date Issued	DEA Registration No.	Name and Address of Registrant
20010101	DEAREGNO	VOID VOID VOID
Schedules		VOID VOID VOID
XXXXXXXXXXXX		VOID VOID VOID
Registered as a	No. of this Order Form	VOID VOID VOID
XXXXXXXXXXXX	000000005	VOID VOID VOID

DEA Form -222
(Oct. 2004) **U.S. OFFICIAL ORDER FORMS - SCHEDULES I & II**
DRUG ENFORCEMENT ADMINISTRATION
SUPPLIER'S Copy 1   107051797

Time needed to complete this activity: 15 minutes

Procedure

On the DEA Form on p. 204:

1. Using a blue or black pen, enter the name of the supplier; the supplier's street address, city, and state; and the date the DEA Form 222 is being filled out.

2. Enter the number of packages, the bottle size, and the name of the medication on the DEA Form 222.

3. Using the *Physicians' Desk Reference* or *Drug Facts and Comparisons,* enter on the DEA Form 222 the NDC number of medications being ordered.

4. Sign the document.

You have been asked to order the following quantities of Schedule II substances for the pharmacy:

- 5 bottles of 100 tablets of Percocet-5
- 1 bottle of 100 tablets of Percodan
- 2 boxes of Duragesic 5 mg
- 4 bottles of 100 tablets of Ritalin 10 mg
- 5 bottles of 100 tablets of Ritalin 5 mg
- 1 bottle of 100 tablets of Ritalin 20 mg
- 2 bottles of 100 capsules of Adderall XR 10 mg
- 3 bottles of 100 tablets of Oxycontin 10 mg
- 1 bottle of 100 tablets of Dilaudid 2 mg

1. The DEA Form 222 is a three-part form; what is done with the three parts of the form?

_____

_____

2. What would you do with a DEA Form 222 if you made an error filling it out?

_____

_____

3. How long must the pharmacy retain a completed DEA Form 222?

_____

_____

Lab Activity #13.2: Receiving a Schedule II order from a wholesaler

Equipment needed:

- Sample DEA Form 222
- *Physicians' Desk Reference* or *Drug Facts and Comparisons*
- Blue ink pen

Time needed to complete this activity: 5 minutes

Directions

The pharmacy has received its order of Schedule II medications that it ordered during the previous activity. The pharmacy has received all of the medications ordered, except that it received 3 bottles of Ritalin 10 mg. Using the DEA Form 222 from the previous activity and a blue pen, complete the remainder of the DEA form.

1. How would you handle the shortage of Ritalin 5 mg?

   _____

   _____

2. Where does a pharmacy keep its Schedule II medications?

   _____

   _____

3. Describe how you would place the medication into stock?

   _____

   _____

   _____

Lab Activity #13.3: Medication recall

Equipment needed:

- Computer with Internet connection
- Paper
- Pen

Time needed to complete this activity: 20 minutes

Procedure

1. Using the Internet, go to *www.fda.gov*.
2. Click on Recalls and Safety Alerts.
3. Answer questions regarding specific medications.

October 9, 2010

1. What strength of Lipitor was recalled?

   _____

2. Why was it recalled?

   _____

3. What should the patient do if he/she has medication being recalled?

   _____

Chapter **13** **Pharmacy Stock and Billing**

September 24, 2010

1. Which company recalled specific lots of Epogen and Procrit?

_____

2. What is Epogen or Procrit indicated to treat?

_____

3. Why were these lots recalled?

_____

4. What NDC numbers were indicated in this drug recall?

_____

_____

_____

_____

_____

_____

July 8, 2010

1. What OTC medications did McNeil Consumer Healthcare recall?

_____

_____

_____

2. Why is the medication being recalled?

_____

_____

3. What telephone number or e-mail address should an individual use to contact McNeil Consumer Healthcare?

_____

_____

Lab Activity #13.4: Define the various types of medication recalls.

Equipment needed:

- Computer with Internet access
- Pencil/pen
- Paper

Time needed to complete this activity: 10 minutes

Procedure

1. Using the Internet, go to *www.fda.gov*.
2. Locate medication recalls
3. Find the definition of Class I, Class II and Class III recalls
1. Define the following terms:

   a. Class I Recall

_____

_____

_____

   b. Class II Recall

_____

_____

_____

   c. Class III Recall

_____

_____

_____

2. What type of Class Recall was involved with Lipitor 40 mg? Why?

_____

_____

_____

3. What type of Class Recall was involved with Epogen and Procrit?

_____

_____

_____

4. What type of Class Recall was involved with McNeil Consumer Healthcare?

_____

_____

_____

Medication Safety and Error Prevention

TERMS AND DEFINITIONS

Select the correct term from the following list and write the corresponding letter in the blank next to the statement.

A. American Society of Health-Care System Pharmacists
B. Automated dispensing systems
C. Medication error prevention
D. Institute for Healthcare Improvements
E. Institute of Medicine
F. Institute for Safe Medication Practices
G. MedWatch
H. National Coordinating Council for Medication Error Reporting and Prevention
I. MedMarx
J. Pharmacy Technician Certification Board
K. Pharmacy Technicians Educators Council
L. United States Pharmacopeia

___E___ 1. Provides scientifically informed analysis and guidance regarding health/health policy

___F___ 2. Organization working toward improvements in health care by promoting promising concepts through safety, efficiency, and other patient-centered goals

___B___ 3. Electronic systems used to dispense medications

___I___ 4. Program for drug and medical product safety alerts and label changes

___D___ 5. Addresses interdisciplinary causes of medication errors and strategies for prevention

___G___ 6. Independent organization that ensures the quality, safety, and benefit of medicines

___J___ 7. Offers national certification for pharmacy technicians in the United States

___K___ 8. Organization that promotes teaching strategies for student instruction

___A___ 9. Association of pharmacists, pharmacy students, and technicians practicing in hospitals and health care systems

___L___ 10. National Internet-accessible database used by hospitals and health care systems

___H___ 11. Devoted entirely to safe medication use and the prevention of medication errors

___C___ 12. Methods used by pharmacy, medicine, nursing, and other health professionals to prevent medication errors

TRUE OR FALSE

Write T or F next to each statement.

___F___ 1. Errors are always caught before they can possibly hurt someone.

___T___ 2. Pharmacy technicians are on the front line when it comes to being able to prevent drug errors.

___T___ 3. Combined sources suggest that as many as 98,000 people per year die from medical errors.

___F___ 4. All drug errors cause harm to the patient.

___T___ 5. One common cause of medication error is illegible handwriting.

___T___ 6. Errors may occur on a weekly basis in many instances.

___T___ 7. Even the most highly skilled person will make errors at one time or another.

___T___ 8. One of the scariest types of error is an error with parenteral medications that take effect quickly.

___True___ 9. Many errors occur as the result of codes on drug products that are not clearly understood.

___T___ 10. Many new systems are in place and are working toward decreasing errors.

___F___ 11. The most important aspect of errors is the reporting process.

Ⓧ ___F___ 12. A drug error cannot be reported anonymously.

___T___ 13. Misinterpreted abbreviations have resulted in drug errors and are an area of concern.

___F___ 14. One of the best ways that errors are decreased is through trial and error.

___T___ 15. It is imperative that every health care worker view drug error prevention as a priority.

MULTIPLE CHOICE

Complete the question by circling the best answer.

1. In 1999 the Institute of Medicine reported that an estimated _____ people per year died from medical errors?
   A. 56,000
   B. 125,000
   C. 44,000
   D. 14,000

2. The 1999 report included errors made by:
   A. Pharmacy staff
   B. Physicians
   C. Nurses
   D. All of the above

3. Which drug was *not* listed in the top 10 medications related to health care professional errors in 2007?
   A. Amoxicillin
   B. Warfarin
   C. Vancomycin
   D. Morphine

4. Most reported medication errors are made in what type of setting?
   A. Hospital pharmacies
   B. Mail order pharmacies
   C. Retail pharmacies
   D. Both A and C

5. Which of the following is *not* an example of the barriers that pharmacy workers face to avoid errors?
   A. Stress
   B. When their lunch hour is
   C. Hard to read labels because of small print
   D. Medication names that sound alike

6. Which of the following is *not* a sound-alike drug?
   A. Bupropion/buspirone
   B. Glipizide/glyburide
   C. Acetaminophen/ibuprofen
   D. Vinblastine/vincristine

7. Anticoagulants such as warfarin have the potential for many interactions with:
   A. Dietary/herbal supplements
   B. Food
   C. Other drugs
   D. All of the above

8. Which of the following drugs is of great concern as a cause of error because it is commonly used to flush IV lines?
   A. Heparin
   B. Saline
   C. Potassium
   D. Dextrose

9. Which of the following abbreviations is not a suffix on a drug label?
   A. LA
   B. DA
   C. ER
   D. SR

10. Receiving care in the home also carries the risk of:
    A. Improper dosing
    B. Contamination of IV sets
    C. High costs
    D. Only A and B

11. Life expectancy in the United States has risen in the last century as the result of:
    A. Improved health care
    B. Increased activity
    C. Better dietary intake
    D. All of the above

12. Many pharmacies fill upward of:
    A. 200 to 300 prescriptions per day
    B. 300 to 400 prescriptions per day
    C. 400 to 500 prescriptions per day
    D. 500 to 600 prescriptions per day

13. The Institute for Healthcare Improvement has reported that more than _____ of all errors in hospitals are due to poor communication of medication orders.
    A. 50%
    B. 45%
    C. 60%
    D. 75%

14. What three steps are involved in medication reconciliation?
    A. Clarification
    B. Verification
    C. Reconciliation
    D. All of the above

15. The ability to prevent mistakes from happening will always fall on people involved in the prescribing, _____, and dosing of medications.
    A. Reading
    B. Writing
    C. Filling
    D. Filing

FILL IN THE BLANK

Answer each question by completing the statement in the space provided.

1. Drug errors are not acceptable in any situation when it comes to _____ _____ and _____.

2. Physicians' handwriting has long been known for its _____ to read.

3. The first response to an error is normally to _____ rather than to _____ the reasons behind such occurrences.

4. No one wants to make an error, but when it does happen, _____ and _____ may emerge.

5. A _____ report can be made to the FDA via the Internet, making it a simple method for reporting a medication error or an adverse event.

SHORT ANSWER

Write a short response to each question in the space provided.

1. Why would a patient try to use medical supplies, intended for single use, more than once, and what risks are associated with this practice?

_____

_____

_____

_____

_____

2. The FDA has recommended new labeling on over-the-counter (OTC) cough and cold medications for children. What does the new label say?

_____

_____

_____

_____

_____

3. What five guidelines are used to share with health care professionals information about potentially dangerous events?

_____

_____

_____

_____

_____

4. What five areas have been outlined by The Joint Commission for patient safety?

_____

_____

_____

_____

_____

5. What are the proposed strategies for safe IV practices?

_____

_____

_____

_____

_____

RESEARCH ACTIVITY

Follow the instructions given in each exercise and provide a response.

1. Access the website at *www.ashp.gov*.

   A. Find and list the guidelines for preventing medication errors in hospitals.

   B. What are the four components regarding the model curriculum for pharmacy technician training?

2. Access the website at *www.ptcb.org*.

   A. What are requirements for certification?

   B. What are continuing education requirements?

CRITICAL THINKING

Reply to each question based on what you have learned in the chapter.

1. An elderly patient has been diagnosed with rheumatoid arthritis. When she is admitted to the hospital, she tells the nurse she takes OTC NSAIDs but cannot remember the names of the medications. Because polypharmacy is a problem with many elderly adults, what steps should be taken by the hospital pharmacy?

   List of all the NSAIDs and ask her which one sounds familiar. It is too risky to go on w/ treatment without knowing what meds the patient takes.

2. Mark is an IV specialist working in a home infusion pharmacy. When he gets an order to prepare a TPN for a 7-year-old girl, he accidentally draws up the strength of the ingredients listed instead of the calculated volumes needed. What will be the consequences if this error is not caught?

   The girl will receive an extremely large volume (concentration) of vitamins and minerals that can potentially have serious and probably fatal consequences.

3. Each individual reacts differently to medications. Metabolism changes occur over time. A technician should pay special attention to the preparation and administration of drugs for the older adult. List three factors that could lead to serious cumulative effects with medications in the elderly. Briefly explain the results of each.

   1- too much blood thinner dosed can cause internal bleeding and eventual death.

   2- Failure to report which meds are taken by the patient can potentially have drastic drug-drug interactions.

   3- There may not be enough strength in the veins for IV dose and we don't want to rupture the patients veins and cause harm.

4. Meticulous care should be taken in the preparation and administration of medications to reduce the chance of error. However, if a mistake is made, how should the technician handle the situation?

   Report the mistake immediately and make sure it is corrected on the floor where the drg administration is taking place. Report to pharmacist. Follow their protocol about how to proceed, depends on severity of error and consequences.

5. James is a pharmacy technician working in a large hospital pharmacy. The critical care nurse calls and asks for the evening dose of daptomycin. She states that the patient is taking the drug q8h. How should James handle this situation?

   Find the physician order for this patient to get proper dosage amounts and routes and tell pharmacist about it. when get the all clear, prepare dose.

6. Brittany is working as an IV technician in a local hospital. She receives a medication order for dopamine for a seriously ill baby on the pediatric floor. The nurse states that it is needed stat. What are the most important factors that Brittany should keep in mind as she prepares the order?

   The concentration of the dose is the most important factor. Must be concentration for infant. Secondly must not contaminate the drug/dose and practice good aseptic technique.

215

LAB SCENARIOS

Pharmacy Abbreviations

Objective: To introduce the pharmacy technician to the many abbreviations encountered in the practice of pharmacy, regardless of the pharmacy setting.

> The pharmacy technician encounters abbreviations when reviewing a prescription/medication order and in pharmacy-related literature. Some of these abbreviations may indicate dosage forms, routes of administration, quantities to be taken, frequency of administration, compounding instructions, and even disease states.
>
> If a pharmacy technician is not familiar with a particular abbreviation, he/she should always ask the pharmacist. The technician should never guess the meaning of an abbreviation. Guessing incorrectly will lead to a medication error and will possibly affect the patient's outcome.
>
> Throughout the years, numerous errors have been associated with misinterpreting abbreviations. As a result of these errors, The Institute of Safe Medication Practices formulated a list of error prone abbreviations, symbols, and dose designations. Many health care organizations have adopted this list, and practitioners within the organization are not to use these abbreviations. However, pharmacy technicians may continue to see them in the community pharmacy setting.

Lab Activity #14.1: Write the meaning of the following pharmaceutical abbreviations.

Equipment needed

- Pen/pencil

Time needed to complete this activity: 20 minutes

PART 1

1. aa _____

2. dtd _____

3. pm _____

4. L _____

5. mcg _____

6. PO _____

7. qh _____

8. supp _____

9. tbsp _____

10. mOsmol _____

11. inj _____

12. gr _____

PART 2

1. ac _____

2. cc _____

3. elix _____

4. kg _____

5. non rep _____

6. noct _____

7. postop _____

8. sol _____

9. top _____

10. ATC _____

11. s _____

12. syr _____

PART 3

1. ad _____

2. caps _____

3. g _____

4. ID _____

5. mEq _____

6. NR _____

7. pr _____

8. susp _____

9. tid _____

10. amp _____

11. bid _____

12. qd _____

Chapter **14** **Medication Safety and Error Prevention**

PART 4

1. ad lib _____

2. c _____

3. Ft _____

4. IM _____

5. mg _____

6. prn _____

7. qs _____

8. tab _____

9. qid _____

10. gtt _____

11. ml _____

12. disp _____

PART 5

1. AM _____

2. BSA _____

3. hs _____

4. IV _____

5. mg/kg _____

6. pulv _____

7. q _____

8. qs ad _____

9. tsp _____

10. aq _____

11. stat _____

12. ung _____

PART 6

1. CA _____

2. EtOH _____

3. KCl _____

4. MVI _____

5. NS _____

6. DW _____

7. O_2 _____

8. H_2O _____

9. LR _____

10. ½ NS _____

11. D5W _____

12. D10W _____

Lab Activity #14.2: Write the organization for each of the following acronyms.

Equipment needed:

• Pencil/pen

Time needed to complete this activity: 5 minutes

1. AAPT _____

2. ACPE _____

3. ASHP _____

4. CDC _____

5. CMS _____

6. CPhT _____

7. DEA _____

8. ExCPT _____

9. FDA _____

10. ISMP _____

11. NABP _____

12. P&T   _____

13. PTCB   _____

14. PTEC   _____

15. TJC   _____

Medication Safety

Objective: To make the pharmacy technician aware that the names of many medications are similar to the names of other medications.

Lab Activity #14.3: Using the ISMP list of commonly confused drug names, identify those medications that are commonly mistaken for the following. (Refer to *www.ismp.org* for the ISMP List of Confused Drug Names for this activity.)

Equipment needed:

- Computer with Internet access
- Pencil/pen

Time needed to complete this activity: 30 minutes

Medication	Mistaken for:
Aciphex	
Actos	
Alkeran	
Amaryl	
aMILoride	
Anacin	
Antivert	
Aricept	
Asacol	
Avandia	
Benicar	
CeleBREX	
Celexa	
Cerebyx	
clonazePAM	
Coumadin	
Cozaar	
DAUNOrubicin	
Diovan	

Medication	Mistaken for:
Effexor	
FLUoxetine	
HumaLOG	
HumuLIN	
Jantoven	
Janumet	
Januvia	
Lasix	
Leukeran	
Levothyroxine	
Lipitor	
Lodine	
LORazepam	
methadone	
Neumega	
Neurontin	
NovoLIN	
Ortho Tri-Cyclen	
Paxil	
Plendil	
predniSONE	
Procanbid	
Tobrex	
Topamax	
Wellbutrin SR	
Yasmin	
Zantac	
Zestril	
Zetia	
Zovirax	
ZyPREXA	

Lab Activity #14.4: Medication errors in the hospital have increased because specific drug classifications and medications are now used. You have been asked to highlight the labels of those medications with a fluorescent pink marker. Indicate whether the following medications should be highlighted. (Refer to *www.ismp.org* for the ISMP List of High-Alert Medications as a reference for this activity.)

Equipment needed:

- Computer with Internet access
- Pencil/pen

Time needed to complete this activity: 15 minutes

Medication	Yes	No
Actoplus Met		
Actos		
Alteplase		
amoxicillin		
Avalide		
Avandia		
cephalexin		
ciprofloxacin		
Digoxin		
Humalog		
Lipitor		
Lovenox		
magnesium sulfate injection		
Metformin		
Novolog Mix 70/30		
oxytocin (IV)		
Plavix		
promethazine (IV)		
sodium chloride for injection (hypertonic)		
total parenteral solutions		
Tricor		
Truvada		
Vytorin		
Warfarin		
Zetia		

Lab Activity #14.5: You are working in a hospital and you have been asked to serve on the Pharmacy and Therapeutics (P&T) Committee. Recently, medication errors due to misinterpretation of pharmacy abbreviations have increased. The P&T committee has been asked to develop a list of approved abbreviations to be used in the hospital. Please indicate whether or not the following abbreviation can be used. If it should not be used, please indicate why. (Refer to *www.ismp.org* for the ISMP List of Error-Prone Abbreviations, Symbols, and Dose Designations.)

Equipment needed:

- Computer with Internet access
- Pencil/pen

Time needed to complete this activity: 15 minutes

Abbreviation	Yes, it may be used	No, it should not be used	If no, why
AD			
Bid			
BT			
Cap			
D/C			
IN			
IU			
OD			
OS			
OU			
qd			
qod			
qhs			
ss			
stat			
Susp			
tab			
tid			
TIW			
U			

Chapter **14** **Medication Safety and Error Prevention**

Lab Activity #14.6: A patient comes to the pharmacy and states that she had difficulty taking the medication and would like to know if she can crush the medication and place it in some applesauce. What would you tell her if she told you she was taking the following medications? (Refer to *www.ismp.org* for ISMP List of Oral Dosage Forms that Should Not Be Crushed.)

Equipment needed:

- Computer with Internet access
- Pencil/pen

Time needed to complete this activity: 20 minutes

Medication	Can it be crushed?	If no, explain
Aciphex		
Actonel		
Amoxicillin tablets		
Bactrim DS		
Boniva		
Cymbalta		
Depakote		
Dyazide		
Erythromycin stearate		
Fosamax		
Hydrea		
Imdur		
Inderal		
Keppra		
Motrin		
Naprosyn		
Nexium		
Oracea		
Paxil		
Ritalin		
Tegretol XR		
Topamax		
Toprol XL		
Xanax		
Zyban		

15 Endocrine System

TERMS AND DEFINITIONS

Select the correct term from the following list and write the corresponding letter in the blank next to the statement.

A. Addison's disease
B. Autoimmune disease
C. Cretinism
D. Cushing's disease
E. Diabetes mellitus
F. Exophthalmos
G. Glucose
H. Goiter
I. Graves' disease
J. Hormones
K. Hypercalcemia
L. Hypocalcemia
M. Hyperglycemia
N. Hypoglycemia
O. Myxedema
P. Osteoporosis
Q. Paget's disease
R. Liothyronine
S. Levothyroxine

_____ 1. Condition in which the development of the brain and body is inhibited by a congenital lack of thyroid secretion

_____ 2. Focal disease of the bone in which the bone structure changes, causing deformity and weakening

_____ 3. Prominence of the eyeball caused by increased thyroid hormone

_____ 4. Abnormally low glucose content circulating in the bloodstream

_____ 5. Condition caused by hypersecretion of thyroid with diffuse goiter, exophthalmos, and skin changes

_____ 6. Unusually high concentration of calcium in the blood

_____ 7. Complex disorder of carbohydrate, fat, and protein metabolism that may result from a deficiency or a complete lack of insulin secretion from cells within the pancreas, or from increased insulin resistance

_____ 8. Simple sugar

_____ 9. Condition resulting in a decrease in adrenocortical hormones, such as mineralocorticoids and glucocorticoids, and the appearance of symptoms such as muscle weakness and weight loss

_____ 10. Low concentration of calcium in the blood

_____ 11. Condition associated with a decrease in bone mass and softening of the bones, resulting in a greater possibility of bone fracture

_____ 12. Known as T_3; contains three ions of iodine

_____ 13. Abnormally high glucose content circulating in the bloodstream

_____ 14. Syndrome that causes increased secretion by the adrenal cortex with excessive production of glucocorticoids, resulting in symptoms such as a moon face and deposits of fat (buffalo hump)

_____ 15. Chemical substances produced and secreted by an endocrine duct into the bloodstream or into another duct, resulting in a physiologic response at a specific target tissue

_____ 16. Condition in which a person's tissues are attacked by the person's own immune system; abnormal antigen–antibody reaction

_____ 17. Condition associated with a decrease in overall thyroid function in adults; also known as hypothyroidism

_____ 18. Condition in which the thyroid is enlarged because of a lack of iodine; known as a simple goiter or, if a tumor is the cause, as a toxic goiter

_____ 19. Known as T_4; contains four iodine ions

225

TRUE OR FALSE

Write T or F next to each statement.

_____ 1. The Greek word for hormone means "to excite."

_____ 2. Hormones control women and their moods only.

_____ 3. All hormones are composed of proteins.

_____ 4. Steroids enter and attach to receptor sites inside the cell.

_____ 5. Melatonin is a chemical substance that helps control the skin's ability to tan.

_____ 6. The pituitary gland is referred to as the *master gland*.

_____ 7. Calcium is the major mineral found in bones.

_____ 8. The pancreas is not the largest organ of the endocrine system.

_____ 9. Men stop producing sperm at some point during their midlife.

_____ 10. The most well-known condition that can affect the pancreas is diabetes.

SYSTEM IDENTIFIER

Identify each organ in this system and enter the term next to the corresponding number.

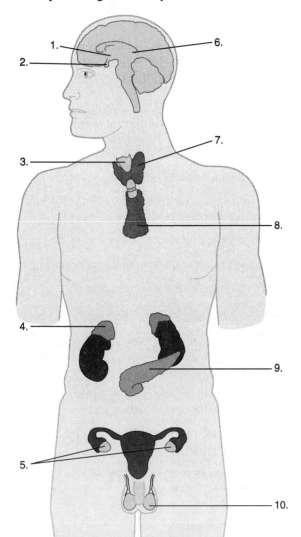

1. _____

2. _____

3. _____

4. _____

5. _____

6. _____

7. _____

8. _____

9. _____

10. _____

MULTIPLE CHOICE

Complete each question by circling the best answer.

1. PTU and methimazole are used for the treatment of:
   A. Diabetes
   B. Osteoporosis
   C. Hyperthyroidism
   D. Estrogen replacement

2. Fosamax and Calcimar are used for the treatment of:
   A. Diabetes
   B. Osteoporosis
   C. Hyperthyroidism
   D. Estrogen replacement

3. The gland that secretes hormones that help the body keep calcium levels adequate is the:
   A. Thyroid
   B. Parathyroid
   C. Hypothalamus
   D. Pituitary

4. The largest endocrine gland is the _____, which produces insulin and glucagon.
   A. Thyroid
   B. Pituitary
   C. Thymus
   D. Pancreas

5. Which of the following is *not* a system that influences the endocrine system?
   A. Positive feedback
   B. Hormonal chemicals that participate in a chain reaction
   C. Negative feedback
   D. Nervous system

6. Which gland influences water balance, body temperature, appetite, and emotions?
   A. Pancreas
   B. Thymus
   C. Thyroid
   D. Hypothalamus

7. Which glands participate in the activities of the kidneys?
   A. Adrenals
   B. Ovaries
   C. Testes
   D. None of the above

8. Failure of the endocrine system to perform correctly affects what area of the body?
   A. Heart
   B. Kidney
   C. Brain
   D. All of the above

9. A goiter is an enlargement of the:
   A. Prostate gland
   B. Pituitary gland
   C. Thyroid gland
   D. Testes

10. Aplasia affects children born without a:
    A. Pineal gland
    B. Pituitary gland
    C. Thyroid gland
    D. Pancreas

11. Conditions such as abnormal uterine bleeding, postmenopausal osteoporosis, and advanced prostate cancer can be treated with:
    A. Estrogen
    B. Progesterone
    C. Testosterone
    D. Insulin

12. Conditions such as certain types of anemia and androgen deficiency can be treated with:
    A. Estrogen
    B. Progesterone
    C. Testosterone
    D. Insulin

FILL IN THE BLANK

Answer each question by completing the statement in the space provided.

1. The _____, _____, and _____ glands, located in the brain, play an important role in hormone production.

2. The _____ is the bridge between the nervous system and the hormone system.

3. _____ hormones act on the cells from which they were secreted, and _____ hormones act on cells near target cells.

4. Two mechanisms of action of glands are _____ and _____.

5. The two different types of hormones in the endocrine system are _____ and _____.

6. The two hormones involved in the "fight or flight reaction" are _____ and _____.

7. The ovaries produce the hormones _____ and _____, and the testes produce

_____.

8. The hormone _____ is responsible for the beginning stages of labor.

9. _____, _____, and _____ are three types of steroids produced in the adrenal cortex.

10. The cause of insulin-dependent diabetes mellitus is the inability of the _____ to produce

_____.

MATCHING

Matching I
Match the drugs with their indications.

_____ 1. Synthroid

_____ 2. Glucophage

_____ 3. Florinef

_____ 4. Prednisone

_____ 5. Aredia

A. Addison's disease
B. Inflammation
C. Thyroid replacement
D. Hypercalcemia
E. Diabetes type 2

Matching II
Match the trade and generic drug names.

_____ 1. Synthroid

_____ 2. Fosamax

_____ 3. Florinef

_____ 4. Premarin

_____ 5. Actos

A. Alendronate
B. Conjugated estrogens
C. Pioglitazone
D. Levothyroxine
E. Fludrocortisone acetate

RESEARCH ACTIVITY

Follow the instructions given in each exercise and provide a response.

1. Access the website *www.nida.nih.gov/infofacts/steroids*. Find information on anabolic steroids that would enable you to answer the following questions:

A. What are they?

B. Who uses them and why?

229

C. What are the side effects?

D. In what controlled substance category are they included?

2. Go to *www.nof.org/osteoporosis/index.* Find out the answers to the following questions:
   A. What is osteoporosis?

   B. The lack of what hormone is a contributing factor?

   C. What are some solutions for osteoporosis?

REFLECT CRITICALLY

CRITICAL THINKING

Reply to each question based on what you have learned in the chapter.

1. Diabetes mellitus (type 2) has been prevalent in your family for the past few years. What lifestyle changes should you make to avoid being diagnosed with this disease?

2. When a young person goes through the adolescence stage of development, the pituitary gland releases hormones that bring about many physical and emotional changes. How many hormones are released, and what parts of the body are affected? What emotional changes take place?

3. The hormone content of meat has been the subject of numerous discussions. Do hormones in meat really affect us physically? If so, how?

RELATE TO PRACTICE

LAB SCENARIOS

Therapeutic Agents for the Endocrine System

Objective: To review with the pharmacy technician the organs of the endocrine system. In addition, to review the brand and generic names, indications, contraindications, adverse effects, dosage forms, routes of administration, and daily dosing of medications used to treat disorders of the endocrine system.

Did You Know?
- 10% of adults 20 years and older suffer from diabetes (diagnosed or undiagnosed).
- Diabetes is the 6th leading cause of death.
- 7.7% of adults 20 years and older are diagnosed with diabetes.
- 2.5% of adults 20 years and older suffer from undiagnosed diabetes.
- 28.6 million ambulatory care visits (to physician office or hospital, outpatient and emergency departments) lead to diabetes as the primary diagnosis.
- 72,449 people die each year as the result of diabetes.

Lab Activity #15.1: Define the following terms associated with the endocrine system.

Equipment needed:

- Medical dictionary
- Pencil/pen

Time needed to complete this activity: 30 minutes

1. Diabetes mellitus

   _____

2. Diabetic neuropathy

   _____

3. Gestational diabetes

   _____

4. Graves' disease

   _____

5. Hashimoto's disease

   _____

6. Hyperglycemia

   _____

7. Hyperthyroidism

_____

8. Hypoglycemia

_____

9. Hypothalamus

_____

10. Hypothyroidism

_____

11. Insulin-dependent diabetes mellitus (IDDM)

_____

12. Insulin resistance

_____

13. Non–insulin-dependent diabetes mellitus (NIDDM)

_____

14. Pancreas

_____

15. Thyroid

_____

Lab Activity #15.2: Using a drug reference book, identify the generic name, drug classification, indications, contraindications, adverse effects, dosage forms, and routes of administration of medications used to treat conditions affecting the endocrine system.

Equipment needed:

- _Drug Facts and Comparisons_ or _Physicians' Desk Reference_
- Pencil/pen

Time needed to complete this activity: 60 minutes

Brand (Trade) Name	Generic Name	Drug Classification	Indication	List Two Contraindications	List Five Adverse Effects	Dosage Forms Available	Routes of Administration	Recommended Daily Dosage
Actoplus Met								
Actos								
Amaryl								
Avandamet								
Avandia								
Cytomel								
Glucophage								
Glucotrol								
Glucovance								
Humalog								
Humalog 70/30								
Humalog Mix 75/25								
Humulin N								
Janumet								

233

Brand (Trade) Name	Generic Name	Drug Classification	Indication	List Two Contraindications	List Five Adverse Effects	Dosage Forms Available	Routes of Administration	Recommended Daily Dosage
Januvia								
Lantus								
Levothyroid								
Levoxyl								
Micronase								
Novolog 70/30								
Prandin								
Precose								
Starlix								
Symlin								
Synthroid								
Tapazole								

16 Nervous System

TERMS AND DEFINITIONS

Select the correct term from the following list and write the corresponding letter in the blank next to the statement.

A. Afferent
B. Autonomic
C. Axon
D. Blood-brain barrier
E. Cell body
F. Cerebrospinal fluid (CSF)
G. Cervical
H. Dendrites
I. Efferent
J. Neurotransmitters
K. Lumbar
L. Monoamine oxidase (MAO)
M. Nerve terminal
N. Neuron
O. Parasympathetic nervous system
P. Peripheral nervous system
Q. Somatic
R. Sympathetic nervous system
S. Thoracic

_____ 1. The motor neurons that control voluntary actions of the skeletal muscles

_____ 2. The main part of a neuron from which axons and dendrites extend

_____ 3. A group of enzymes (includes MAO-A and MAO-B) found in the nerve terminals and liver cells; inactivates chemicals such as tyramine, catecholamines, serotonin, and certain medications

_____ 4. The segment of a neuron that branches out to bring impulses to the cell body

_____ 5. The conduction of electrical impulses away from the central nervous system (CNS) of the body

_____ 6. The part of a nerve cell that conducts impulses away from the cell body

_____ 7. The region of the back that includes the area between the ribs and the pelvis; the area around the waist

_____ 8. Division of the autonomic nervous system (ANS) that functions during restful situations; the "breed or feed" part of the ANS

_____ 9. Chemicals that are transmitted from one neuron to another as electrical nerve impulses

_____10. Relates to the area of the thorax or the chest

_____11. A fluid that fills the ventricles of the brain and also lies in the space between the arachnoid layer of the meninges, brain, or spinal cord

_____12. The functional unit of the nervous system that includes the cell body, dendrites, axons, and terminals

_____13. The end portion of the neuron in which nerve impulses cause chemicals to be released; these cross a small space called a *synaptic cleft* to carry the impulse to another neuron

_____14. Division of the ANS that functions during stressful situations; the "flight or fight" part of the ANS

_____15. Self-controlling or involuntary

_____16. Division of the nervous system outside the brain and spinal cord

_____17. A barrier formed by special characteristics of capillaries that prevents certain chemicals from moving into the brain

_____18. The direction of neuronal impulses from the body toward the CNS

_____19. The neck region

TRUE OR FALSE

Write T or F next to each statement.

_____ 1. The human nervous system is a simple body system.

_____ 2. The CNS consists of the brain and spinal cord.

_____ 3. The nerve impulses are transmitted by various chemicals called *neurotransmitters*.

_____ 4. Most drugs that can pass through the blood-brain barrier are water soluble.

_____ 5. The somatic nervous system is part of the CNS.

_____ 6. Sympathetic and parasympathetic systems are part of the ANS.

_____ 7. Individuals with Parkinson's disease have low levels of dopamine.

_____ 8. Few differences can be found between the sympathetic and parasympathetic systems.

_____ 9. Most indications for skeletal muscle relaxants are for short-term use.

_____10. Patients with epilepsy need to take their medication only after a seizure.

MULTIPLE CHOICE

Complete each question by circling the best answer.

1. The smallest functional part of the CNS is the:
   A. Brain
   B. Synapse
   C. Spinal cord
   D. Neuron

2. The largest area of the brain is the:
   A. Cerebral cortex
   B. Cerebellum
   C. Thalamus
   D. Hypothalamus

3. The midbrain, pons, and medulla oblongata are all part of the:
   A. Cerebrum
   B. Brainstem
   C. Cerebellum
   D. Spinal cord

4. Which of the following is *not* a main neurotransmitter of the sympathetic system?
   A. Dopamine
   B. Epinephrine
   C. Acetylcholine
   D. Norepinephrine

5. A patient suffering from premature labor could be given:
   A. Levophed
   B. Intropin
   C. Terbutaline
   D. Pitocin

6. Dry mouth and inhibition of urine output are side effects of:
   A. Sympathomimetics
   B. Anticholinergics
   C. Adrenergics
   D. Parasympathomimetics

7. Which of the following is *not* a generalized seizure?
   A. Petit mal
   B. Status epilepticus
   C. Tonic-clonic
   D. None of the above

8. Besides taking their medications, individuals with epilepsy may be able to help themselves by:
   A. Learning relaxation techniques
   B. Avoiding flashing lights
   C. A and B
   D. None of the above

9. An abnormal loss of memory and basic mental function is called:
   A. Epilepsy
   B. Dementia
   C. Seizures
   D. Blood-brain barrier

10. A condition associated with loss or a deficiency of dopamine is:
    A. Alzheimer's disease
    B. Parkinson's disease
    C. Multiple sclerosis
    D. Lou Gehrig's disease

FILL IN THE BLANK

Answer each question by completing the statement in the space provided.

1. The three main states of a neuron are _____, _____, and
   _____.

2. The hypothalamus is a _____ and _____.

3. The thin covering that protects the brain and spinal cord from the bony structures of the skull and spinal
   column is the _____.

4. The two branches of the PNS are called the _____ and _____ nervous
   systems, which regulate _____ and _____ _____.

5. Drugs that mimic the actions of the sympathetic nervous system are called _____
   _____ and drugs that mimic the parasympathetic nervous system are called
   _____.

6. Alpha receptors are located on _____ _____;
   beta$_1$-receptors are located on the _____, and beta$_2$-receptors are located in the
   _____ _____ and elsewhere.

7. The function of the sympathetic division is to respond to _____ situations; one of the main
   functions of the parasympathetic system is to activate the _____ system.

8. The main neurotransmitters of the sympathetic system are _____ and _____,
   and the main neurotransmitter of the parasympathetic system is _____.

9. The two main types of skeletal muscle relaxants are _____ acting and _____
   acting.

10. The main class of drugs used to treat myasthenia gravis is _____.

MATCHING

Matching I

Match the following disease states with their drug treatment classes.

_____ 1. Epilepsy

_____ 2. Alzheimer's disease

_____ 3. Multiple sclerosis

_____ 4. Parkinson's disease

_____ 5. Amyotrophic lateral sclerosis (ALS)

A. Autoimmune stimulants (interferons)
B. Dopamine-increasing drugs
C. Cholinesterase inhibitors
D. Riluzole
E. Anticonvulsants

Matching II

Match the following drugs with the diseases they treat.

_____ 1. Phenytoin

_____ 2. Aricept

_____ 3. Avonex

_____ 4. Sinemet

_____ 5. Mestinon

A. Parkinson's disease
B. Myasthenia gravis
C. Alzheimer's disease
D. Epilepsy
E. Multiple sclerosis

SHORT ANSWER

Write a short response to each question in the space provided.

1. What are the most common symptoms of Parkinson's disease?

_____

_____

2. What happens to the brain cells in a patient with Alzheimer's disease?

_____

_____

3. Name four drug therapies used in the treatment of seizures.

_____

_____

RESEARCH ACTIVITY

Follow the instructions given in each exercise and provide a response.

1. Access the website *http://en.wikipedia.org/wiki/caffeine* and answer the following questions:
   A. Where is caffeine found in nature?

   B. How does it affect the nervous system?

2. Access *www.nida.nih.gov/Alzheimers/publications/medication.html*. Find and list the latest drugs approved for the treatment of Alzheimer's disease.

REFLECT CRITICALLY

CRITICAL THINKING

Reply to each question based on what you have learned in the chapter.

1. It is said that geniuses use approximately 10% of their brain capacity.
   A. About what percentage does the average person use?

   B. What activities can one do to create neuronal connections in the brain?

239

C. What is the meaning of the saying, "If you don't use it, you'll lose it"?

2. Many people experience a "rush of adrenaline" or a "natural high" from participating in dangerous sports. What does this mean, and what part of the nervous system is affected?

3. You are suddenly called on in class to make a short oral presentation. Describe what mental and emotional changes are taking place in your mind and body as you prepare to carry out your assignment.

4. How is the blood-brain barrier like a fence around your home?

17 Psychopharmacology

TERMS AND DEFINITIONS

Select the correct term from the following list and write the corresponding letter in the blank next to the statement.

A. Attention deficit hyperactivity disorder (ADHD)
B. Cognition
C. Depression
D. Dystonia
E. Extrapyramidal symptoms
F. Insomnia
G. Mania
H. Neurosis
I. Phobias
J. Psychosis
K. Schizophrenia
L. Tardive dyskinesia
M. Psychotherapy

_L_ 1. Symptoms that include twisting, repeated jerking movements, and/or abnormal posture

_E_ 2. Side effects of antipsychotic medications; symptoms include parkinsonism, dystonias, and tremors

_I_ 3. Continuous irrational fear of a thing, place, or situation that causes significant distress

_B_ 4. Activities associated with thinking, learning, and memory

_G_ 5. A form of psychosis characterized by excessive excitement, elevated moods, and exalted feelings

_M_ 6. Professional therapy that includes helping the patient work through personal problems that affect emotions and behaviors

_A_ 7. Physiological brain disorder that affects the ability to engage in quiet, passive activities or to focus one's attention due to an imbalance of neurotransmitters in the brain

_C_ 8. A mental state characterized by sadness, a feeling of loss, grief, loss of appetite, and possibly suicidal thoughts

_J_ 9. A mental illness characterized by loss of contact with reality

_D_ 10. Unwanted side effects of treatment with phenothiazines, including slow, rhythmical, involuntary movements that are either generalized or specific to a muscle group

_K_ 11. A group of mental disorders characterized by inappropriate emotions and unrealistic thinking

_H_ 12. Mental illness, without loss of contact with reality, arising from stress or anxiety factors in the patient's environment; phobias can be listed in this category

_F_ 13. Difficulty falling or staying asleep

TRUE OR FALSE

Write T or F next to each statement.

___T___ 1. Because of the brain's complexity, the study of the brain is one of the most difficult disciplines in medicine.

___F___ 2. Psychologists can write prescriptions for mental health disorders.

___F___ 3. The nervous system is an intricate network of bones and muscles.

___T___ 4. Because of the wide range of mental conditions, many choices for treatment are available.

___T___ 5. Everyone suffers from depression at some time.

___T___ 6. Patients with bipolar disorder are commonly called *manic-depressives*.

___F___ 7. Tricyclic antidepressants (TCAs), monoamine oxidase inhibitors (MAOIs), and selective serotonin reuptake inhibitors (SSRIs) may be taken concurrently when taken for depression.

___T___ 8. TCAs are not the first line of treatment for depression.

___F___ 9. It is estimated that 10% to 25% of the population have insomnia.

___T___ 10. ADHD symptoms and signs include impulsive, explosive, or irritable behavior.

MULTIPLE CHOICE

Complete each question by circling the best answer.

1. Which of the following is **not** an antipsychotic agent?
   A. Haldol
   B. Desyrel — antidepressant
   C. Risperdal
   D. Zyprexa

2. Traditionally, mentally ill patients were treated with:
   A. Electric shock
   B. Straightjackets
   C. Isolation
   D. A, B, and C

3. The field of psychology is the study of:
   A. Human behavior
   B. Human emotions
   C. Human behavior and emotions
   D. Human emotions, feelings, and behavior

4. Which of the following is **not** a specialist in the field of mental health?
   A. Psychiatrist
   B. Counselor
   C. Bartender
   D. Psychologist

5. Which of the following is **not** an example of group therapy?
   A. Confessional
   B. Alcoholics Anonymous
   C. Weight Watchers
   D. Narcotics Anonymous

6. Which mental health specialist(s) can write prescriptions?
   - A. Psychologist
   - B. Psychiatrist
   - C. Neurologist
   - **D.** B and C

7. Schizophrenia, mania, and psychotic depression can be treated with:
   - **A.** Antipsychotics
   - **B.** Antidepressants
   - C. Tranquilizers
   - D. All of the above

8. Elavil, Sinequan, and Tofranil are all examples of:
   - A. Antipsychotics
   - **B.** Antidepressants
   - C. Antianxiety agents
   - D. Insomnia agents

9. Which class of antidepressants can be prescribed for chronic pain?
   - **A.** TCAs
   - B. MAOIs
   - C. SSRIs
   - D. OTCs

10. Which class of drug interacts with many foods and OTC agents?
    - A. TCAs
    - **B.** MAOIs
    - C. SSRIs
    - D. MOAs

11. Paxil, Prozac, and Zoloft are all examples of:
    - A. TCAs
    - B. MAOIs
    - **C.** SSRIs
    - D. OTCs

12. Which two types of drugs must not be taken together?
    - A. TCAs and MAOIs
    - B. TCAs and SSRIs
    - **C.** MAOIs and SSRIs
    - D. None of the above

13. The drug bupropion ~wellbutrin~ is indicated for _____ in addition to depression.
    - A. Weight loss
    - **B.** Smoking cessation
    - C. Alcohol withdrawal
    - D. Hiccup relief

14. Antipsychotics, antidepressants, antianxiety drugs, and benzodiazepines should all have which auxiliary label?
    A. Take at bedtime
    B. Take with food
    C. Avoid dairy products
    D. May cause drowsiness and dizziness

15. Imipramine is indicated for enuresis, which is:
    A. An eating disorder
    B. Insomnia
    C. Bedwetting
    D. Loss of hair

16. The most common ingredient in OTC sleep aids is:
    A. Diphenhydrinate
    B. Diphenhydramine
    C. Acetaminophen
    D. Digoxin

FILL IN THE BLANK

Answer each question by completing the statement in the space provided.

1. Depression can be treated effectively in most cases using _____ and/or _____ medications.

2. _____ is the oldest prescription agent used to treat the mania phase of bipolar disorder.

3. The four closely related medication classes used to treat depression are _____,
   _____, _____, and _____.

4. There are several agents used to treat depression by affecting _____ _____.

5. OTC sedatives are used to treat _____ _____ insomnia
   and _____ _____.

6. _____ are still used in many hospitals as _____ for surgery.

7. _____ can be expressed as a feeling of fear or dread.

8. The two side effects of antipsychotic agents are _____ and _____.

9. MAOIs react with foods containing _____, which can cause a dangerous increase in
   _____ _____.

10. The brain is protected by the _____ _____ _____, which
    prevents many _____ from passing into it.

MATCHING

Matching I

Match the drug classifications with their indications.

___D___ 1. Phenothiazines

___C___ 2. Hypnotics

___E___ 3. MAOIs

___B___ 4. SSRIs

___A___ 5. Sedatives

A. Agents that induce sleep
B. Preferable treatment for depression and obsessive compulsive disorder (OCD)
C. Used to relax a nervous or irritated person
D. Treat psychosis, or nausea, and vomiting
E. Can cause hypertension

Matching II

Match the drugs with their classifications.

___C___ 1. Haldol

___E___ 2. Celexa

___A___ 3. Phenobarbital

___B___ 4. Xanax

___D___ 5. Ambien

A. Sedative (barbiturate)
B. Antianxiety agent
C. Antipsychotic
D. Hypnotic
E. SSRI antidepressant

Matching III

Match the following trade and generic drug names.

___C___ 1. Valium

___E___ 2. Zoloft

___A___ 3. Elavil

___B___ 4. Risperdal

___D___ 5. Compazine

A. Amitriptyline
B. Risperidone
C. Diazepam
D. Prochlorperazine
E. Sertraline

RESEARCH ACTIVITY

Follow the instructions given in each exercise and provide a response.

1. Access the website *http://en.wikipedia.org/wiki/psychopharmacology*
   A. Read the history section.

   B. What is the connection between opioids and psychotropic drugs?

2. Access the website *www.nida.nih.gov/infofacts/Ritalin.html*
   A. How does Ritalin work?

B. What neurotransmitter in the brain does it affect?

C. Is it really effective against ADHD?

REFLECT CRITICALLY

CRITICAL THINKING

Reply to each question based on what you have learned in the chapter.

1. Give three reasons so many people are becoming addicted to prescription drugs.

   1- People are paranoid there is something wrong with them and so get prescribed a drug they do not even need.

   2- People want the quick fix of drugs and do not change lifestyle so depend solely on drug for alleviation.

   3- Doctors are prescribing addictive drugs with the intention to help a patient, instead of forcing (how?) a lifestyle change.

2. What is contributing to the rise in attention deficit disorder (ADD)/ADHD/OCD in children? Does it have anything to do with preservatives or hormones in food?

   The speed of technology is much faster now. Kids are coming into this world w/ terabytes of information available at their fingertips. To even scratch the surface, we must be very fast in all we do. It is a direct cause of the need for speed and demand of fast results, fast food, everything fast. Probably has nothing to do w/ food, but maybe.

3. When a person is categorized as "neurotic" and a "hypochondriac," what exactly does this mean? Do you think there is any "cure" for those conditions? Are they real psychological conditions that can be treated?

   It is just people who more or less obsess over specific, usually negative, things. The "cure" is probably just an understanding of their thinking patterns and deepening ability to catch themselves going down a neurotic thought-chain. Self-knowledge is key.

LAB SCENARIOS

Therapeutic Agents for the Nervous System

Objective: To review with the pharmacy technician terms associated with the nervous system and review the brand and generic names, indication, contraindications, adverse effects, dosage forms, routes of administration, and recommended daily dosage of medications used to treat disorders of the nervous system.

DID YOU KNOW?
- Epilepsy affects about 2.5 million Americans.
- About 10% of people will experience a seizure at some point during their lifetime, and about 3% will have had a diagnosis of epilepsy by the age of 80.
- In 2009, nearly 150,000 new cases of epilepsy will be diagnosed in the United States.
- Epilepsy results in an estimated annual cost of $15.5 billion in medical costs and lost or reduced earnings and production.
- 8.5 million ambulatory care visits (to physician offices or hospital outpatient and emergency departments) with major depression as the primary diagnosis.
- 3.1% of adults have been diagnosed with serious psychological distress in the past 30 days.
- In 2006, there were 55.7 million ambulatory care visits with mental disorders as the primary diagnosis.
- 5.0 million (8%) of children 3 to 17 years of age are diagnosed with ADHD.
- 11% of all boys 3 to 17 years of age are diagnosed with ADHD.

Lab Activity #17.1: Define the following terms associated with the nervous system.

Equipment needed:

- Medical dictionary
- Pencil/pen

Time needed to complete this activity: 30 minutes.

1. Absence seizures _____

2. Alzheimer's disease _____

3. Anxiety disorder _____

4. ADHD _____

5. Bipolar disease _____

6. Cluster headache _____

7. Convulsion _____

8. Dementia _____

9. Depression _____

10. Epilepsy _____

11. Focal seizures _____

12. Inflammation _____

13. Insomnia _____

14. Mania _____

15. Migraine _____

16. Myoclonic seizures _____

17. Narcolepsy _____

18. Neuropathic pain _____

19. OCD _____

20. Panic disorder _____

21. Parkinson's disease _____

22. Petit mal seizures _____

23. Phobia _____

24. Posttraumatic stress disorder (PTSD) _____

25. Psychoses _____

26. Schizophrenia _____

27. Status epilepticus _____

28. Tonic-clonic seizures _____

Lab Activity #17.2: Using a drug reference book, identify the generic name, drug classification, indication, contraindications, adverse effects, dosage forms, routes of administration, and recommended daily dosage of medications used to treat conditions affecting the nervous system.

Equipment needed:

▪ *Drug Facts & Comparisons* or *Physicians' Desk Reference*
▪ Pencil/pen

Time needed to complete this activity: 60 minutes.

Brand (Trade) Name	Generic Name	Drug Classification	Indication	List Two Contraindications	List Five Adverse Effects	Dosage Forms Available	Routes of Administration	Recommended Daily Dosage
Abilify								
Actiq								
Adderall XR								
Ambien CR								
Anaprox								
Aricept								
Ativan								
Budeprion SR								
Budeprion XL								
Buprenex								
BuSpar								
Celebrex								
Celexa								
Clozaril								
Cogentin								
Concerta								
Cymbalta								
Daypro								

Continued

Brand (Trade) Name	Generic Name	Drug Classification	Indication	List Two Contraindications	List Five Adverse Effects	Dosage Forms Available	Routes of Administration	Recommended Daily Dosage
Depakote								
Depakote ER								
Desyrel								
Dilantin								
Duragesic								
Effexor XR								
Endocet								
Focalin XR								
Geodon								
Imitrex								
Keppra								
Klonopin								
Lamictal								
Lexapro								
Lithonate								
Lunesta								
Lyrica								

Maxalt							
Maxalt ML							
Mirapex							
Motrin							
Mysoline							
Namenda							
Naproxen							
OxyContin							
Paxil							
Provigil							
Prozac							
Relafen							
Relpax							
Remeron							
Requip							
Risperdal							
Risperdal Consta							
Seroquel							

Continued

Brand (Trade) Name	Generic Name	Drug Classification	Indication	List Two Contraindications	List Five Adverse Effects	Dosage Forms Available	Routes of Administration	Recommended Daily Dosage
Sinequan								
Strattera								
Suboxone								
Symmetrel								
Tegretol								
Topamax								
Toradol								
Trileptal								
Tylenol with Codeine								
Ultram ER								
Vicodin								
Vicoprofen								
Wellbutrin XL								
Xanax								
Zoloft								
Zomig								
Zonegran								
Zyprexa								

18 Respiratory System

TERMS AND DEFINITIONS

Select the correct term from the following list and write the corresponding letter in the blank next to the statement.

A. Asthma
B. Chronic obstructive pulmonary disease (COPD)
C. Cough reflex
D. Cystic fibrosis (CF)
E. Decongestant
F. Expectorant
G. Influenza
H. Metered dose inhaler (MDI)
I. Nonproductive cough
J. Productive cough
K. Prophylaxis
L. Sputum
M. Viscosity
N. Antitussive

_____ 1. Fluid coughed up from the lungs and bronchial tissues

_____ 2. The thickness of a solution or fluid (e.g., corn syrup is very viscous)

_____ 3. Response of the body intended to clear air passages of foreign substances and mucus by forceful expiration

_____ 4. An inherited disorder that causes production of very thick mucus in the respiratory tract and that affects the pancreas and sweat glands

_____ 5. Medication that prevents or relieves coughing

_____ 6. A method of supplying medication to the lungs through a pressurized inhalation

_____ 7. A respiratory tract infection caused by an influenza virus

_____ 8. Drugs that reduce swelling of the mucous membranes by constricting dilated blood vessels, diminishing blood flow to nasal tissues, and thereby reducing nasal congestion

_____ 9. Cough that expectorates mucous secretions from the respiratory tract

_____ 10. A disease process in which the lungs have a decreased capacity for gas exchange; two types are *emphysema* and *chronic bronchitis*

_____ 11. Preventive treatment

_____ 12. Chemical that aids the removal of mucous secretions from the respiratory system by loosening and thinning sputum and bronchial secretions

_____ 13. A condition in which inflammation and narrowing of the airways impedes breathing

_____ 14. Cough that does not produce mucous secretions (dry cough)

TRUE OR FALSE

Write T or F next to each statement.

_____ 1. The respiratory rates of a child and an adult are the same.

_____ 2. Cartilage around the larynx is usually only visible in men.

_____ 3. The left bronchus is bigger than the right bronchus.

_____ 4. The diaphragm separates the chest cavity from the abdominal area.

_____ 5. Breathing is an involuntary mechanism.

_____ 6. When a person has pneumonia, the condition always affects only one lung.

_____ 7. Older adults are at a high risk for pneumonia, especially after an injury.

_____ 8. Asthma is classified as an inflammatory lung disease.

_____ 9. Tuberculosis is the most common bacterial disease affecting the pulmonary system worldwide.

_____10. Individuals who have high blood pressure should take Sudafed regularly.

SYSTEM IDENTIFIER

Identify each anatomical part in this system and enter the term next to the corresponding number.

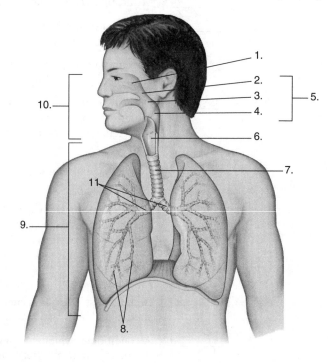

1. _____   7. _____

2. _____   8. _____

3. _____   9. _____

4. _____   10. _____

5. _____   11. _____

6. _____

254

MULTIPLE CHOICE

Complete each question by circling the best answer.

1. The body's pH level must remain close to:
   A. 1.7
   B. 5.6
   C. 6.5
   D. 7.4

2. Where does the exchange of gases take place?
   A. Trachea
   B. Bronchi
   C. Bronchioles
   D. Alveolar sacs

3. Which of the following is *not* a part of the upper respiratory system?
   A. Trachea
   B. Larynx
   C. Pharynx
   D. Nose

4. The windpipe is called the:
   A. Trachea
   B. Larynx
   C. Pharynx
   D. Nose

5. The voice box is called the:
   A. Trachea
   B. Larynx
   C. Pharynx
   D. Nose

6. Which of the following is *not* a part of the lower respiratory tract?
   A. Larynx
   B. Trachea
   C. Bronchioles
   D. Lungs

7. To relieve a dry, nonproductive cough and to loosen mucus so that it can be expelled through coughing, a patient can take a (an):
   A. Antitussive
   B. Expectorant
   C. Antihistamine
   D. Decongestant

8. Dyspnea is a condition characterized by:
   A. Respiration stops
   B. Rapid breathing
   C. Labored or difficult breathing
   D. Lack of breathing that causes the skin to turn blue-gray

9. *Rhinorrhea* is the medical name for a (an):
   A. Allergy
   B. Cold
   C. Sore throat
   D. Runny nose

10. Emphysema can be caused by:
    A. Repeated bronchial infections
    B. Smoking
    C. Genetic disposition
    D. All of the above

FILL IN THE BLANK

Answer each question by completing the statement in the space provided.

1. The act of respiration is broken down into the two distinct phases of _____ and _____.

2. During inspiration, the diaphragm _____, the intercostals _____, and the size of the thoracic cavity _____.

3. The functions of nasal mucous membranes are to _____ and _____ inhaled air.

4. The function of bronchioles is to provide _____ distribution and passageways for _____ to reach the alveoli.

5. The main function of the lungs is breathing, also known as _____ _____.

6. The respiratory control center is located in the _____ of the brain.

7. The three mechanisms that cause a person to sneeze are _____ _____, _____ _____, and _____ _____.

8. Two common treatments for the symptoms of a cold are _____ and _____.

9. The vaccine that gives immunity for 14 common strains of *S. pneumoniae* respiratory infections is _____.

10. Three treatments for bronchitis, emphysema, and asthma are _____, _____, and _____.

MATCHING

Matching I
Match the following classes of drugs with their mechanisms of action.

_____ 1. Antitussives

_____ 2. Mucolytics

_____ 3. Decongestant

_____ 4. Corticosteroids

_____ 5. Anticholinergics

A. Help clear respiratory passages
B. Act as antiinflammatory agents
C. Break up mucus in patients with COPD and CF
D. Inhibit the action of acetylcholine (Ach)
E. Suppress coughing

Matching II
Match the disease states with their drug treatments.

_____ 1. Tuberculosis (TB)

_____ 2. Chronic asthma

_____ 3. Cold

_____ 4. COPD

_____ 5. Cough

A. Pseudoephedrine
B. Guaifenesin
C. Isoniazid
D. Triamcinolone inhalation
E. Ipratropium inhalation

RESEARCH ACTIVITY

Follow the instructions given in each exercise and provide a response.

1. Visit the website *http://www.lungusa.org*. Type the words "secondhand smoke" in the search bar. Read about secondhand smoke and its effects on children.

2. Access the website *www.cdc.gov*. Read the information found under Avian flu virus—Key facts.

3. Access the website *http://www.nlm.nih.gov/medlineplus/cysticfibrosis.html*. Read the information about CF. Whom does this disease affect? What are some of the physical difficulties patients with CF encounter?

CRITICAL THINKING

Reply to each question based on what you have learned in the chapter.

1. Smoking has increased dramatically among teenagers over the years. What do you think has been a contributing factor to the increase?

2. What are the health benefits of having plants in your home and office?

3. While having dinner in a restaurant, you see a person who may be choking. You quickly go over to help. What is the first question you should ask the person? Why?

4. Pseudoephedrine now must be sold by a pharmacist, and customers must fill out a log book for their purchase. Why is the sale of pseudoephedrine now controlled?

5. Why do some people become ill with the flu even if they have received the flu vaccine?

LAB SCENARIOS

Therapeutic Agents for the Respiratory System

Objective: To review with the pharmacy technician terms associated with the respiratory system and review the brand and generic names, indication, contraindications, adverse effects, dosage forms, routes of administration, and recommended daily dosage of medications used to treat disorders of the respiratory system.

DID YOU KNOW?
- 9.8 million (4.4%) adults were diagnosed with chronic bronchitis in the past year.
- 3.8 million (1.7%) adults have been diagnosed with emphysema.
- 7 million (9.4%) children have asthma in the United States.
- 16.4 million (7.3%) adults suffer from asthma.
- 10.6 million visits are made to office-based physicians each year to treat asthma.

Lab Activity #18.1: Define the following terms associated with the respiratory system

Equipment needed:

- Medical dictionary
- Pencil/pen

Time needed to complete this activity: 15 minutes.

1. Allergic asthma _____

2. Allergic rhinitis _____

3. Anaphylaxis _____

4. Asthma _____

5. Bronchitis _____

6. COPD _____

7. Emphysema _____

Lab Activity #18.2: Using a drug reference book, identify the generic name, drug classification, indication, contraindications, adverse effects, dosage forms, routes of administration, and recommended daily dosage of medications used to treat conditions affecting the respiratory system.

Equipment needed:

- *Drug Facts & Comparisons or Physicians' Desk Reference*
- Pencil/pen

Time needed to complete this activity: 45 minutes

Brand (Trade) Name	Generic Name	Drug Classification	Indication	List Two Contraindications	List Five Adverse Effects	Dosage Forms Available	Routes of Administration	Recommended Daily Dosage
Accolate								
Advair Diskus								
Allegra-D 12 Hour								
Allegra-D 24 Hour								
Astelin								
Azmacort								
Clarinex								
Combivent								
Flonase								
Flovent HFA								
Nasacort AQ								
Nasarel								

Nasonex	ProAir HFA	Proventil HFA	Pulmicort Respules	Rhinocort AQ	Serevent	Singulair	Spiriva	Symbicort	Ventolin	Xopenex	Xopenex HFA	Zyflo	

TERMS AND DEFINITIONS

Select the correct term from the following list and write the corresponding letter in the blank next to the statement.

A. Accommodation
B. Acoustic nerve
C. Aqueous humor
D. Auditory canal
E. Auditory ossicles
F. Cataract
G. Cones
H. Cornea
I. Conjunctiva
J. Eustachian tube
K. Labyrinth
L. Miosis
M. Mydriasis
N. Orbit
O. Ophthalmic
P. Otic
Q. Rods
R. Tympanic membrane

_____ 1. The transparent tissue covering the anterior portion of the eye

_____ 2. Pertaining to the ear

_____ 3. Bony maze composed of vestibule, cochlea, and semicircular canals of the inner ear

_____ 4. Dilation of the pupil

_____ 5. Pertaining to the eye

_____ 6. Photoreceptors responsible for color (daylight vision)

_____ 7. Transparent protective mucous membrane that lines the underside of the eyelid

_____ 8. A 1-inch segment of tube that runs from the external ear to the middle ear

_____ 9. A membranous skin that separates the external ear from the middle ear

_____ 10. Eye socket

_____ 11. Contraction of the pupil

_____ 12. Photoreceptors responsible for black and white colors that respond to dim light

_____ 13. The set of three small, bony structures in the ear (i.e., the malleus, incus, and stapes)

_____ 14. The fluid found in the anterior and posterior chambers of the eye

_____ 15. The change that occurs in the ocular lens when it focuses at various distances

_____ 16. Loss of transparency of the lens of the eye

_____ 17. A tubular structure in the middle ear that runs to the nasopharynx (throat)

_____ 18. The cranial nerve that controls the senses of hearing and equilibrium and that eventually leads to the cerebellum and the medulla

TRUE OR FALSE

Write T or F next to each statement.

_____ 1. The cornea contains blood vessels that provide nourishment to the eye.

_____ 2. The iris is responsible for the color of the eye.

_____ 3. Glaucoma can cause blindness.

_____ 4. About 90% of individuals with glaucoma have open-angle glaucoma.

_____ 5. Lacrimal glands are activated by the sympathetic nervous system.

_____ 6. Ophthalmic erythromycin comes in many dosage forms.

_____ 7. The eustachian tube is located in the middle ear.

_____ 8. The human ear is only responsible for hearing.

_____ 9. An ophthalmic medication commonly is prescribed to treat an otic condition.

_____10. Most infections of the ear are caused by bacterial infections.

MULTIPLE CHOICE

Complete each question by circling the best answer.

1. Alteration of which two senses can most dramatically change a life?
   A. Sight and touch
   B. Smell and taste
   C. Hearing and sight
   D. Smell and hearing

2. A person who is trained to perform an eye examination is called an:
   A. Optician
   B. Optometrist
   C. Optimist
   D. Ophthalmologist

3. The purpose of the eyebrow is to:
   A. Make the eye more attractive
   B. Trap sweat
   C. Help keep the eyes moist
   D. Shade the eyes from light

4. The lateral rectus rotates:
   A. Outward
   B. Inward
   C. Upward and outward
   D. Downward and inward

5. Glaucoma is caused by:
   A. Viral infections
   B. Bacterial infections
   C. Increased pressure within the eye
   D. Allergies

6. Which of the following is not a cause of conjunctivitis?
   A. Virus
   B. Bacterial infections
   C. Increased pressure within the eye
   D. Allergies

7. Which drug would be indicated for glaucoma?
   A. Ciloxan
   B. Timoptic
   C. Genoptic
   D. Viroptic

8. A possible side effect of Xalatan is:
   A. Drowsiness
   B. Nausea and vomiting
   C. Diarrhea
   D. Changes in iris color

9. What are the two major functions of the eardrum?
   A. To produce cerumen
   B. To protect the middle ear from foreign objects
   C. To transmit sound toward the middle ear
   D. B and C

10. A ringing or buzzing in the ear is called:
    A. Tinnitus
    B. Tendonitis
    C. Rhinitis
    D. Conjunctivitis

11. The part of the eye that contains the enzyme lysozyme and that has antimicrobial properties is the:
    A. Retina
    B. Sclera
    C. Lacrimal gland (tears)
    D. Conjunctiva

12. The _____ contain(s) the photoreceptive cells for vision.
    A. Choroids
    B. Cornea
    C. Vitreous body
    D. Retina

FILL IN THE BLANK

Answer each question by completing the statement in the space provided.

1. An alternative to wearing glasses is _____ surgery.

2. Two new treatments to reverse the effects of blindness are _____ _____ and
   _____ _____ .

3. Three common ophthalmic dosage forms are _____, _____, and
   _____.

4. Carbonic anhydrase inhibitors (CAIs) are used as a long-term treatment for _____
   _____ _____, whereas miotics are used only preoperatively for individuals
   with _____ _____ _____.

5. Most of the agents used to reduce inflammation of the eyes or the ears are _____ and
   _____ (dosage forms).

6. Decongestants and antihistamines are used to combat _____.

7. Three common viral infections of the eye are _____, _____, and
   _____.

8. The three main functions of the ear are _____, _____, and
   _____.

9. The fluid-filled inner ear is called the _____; it transmits sound via _____ to the brain.

10. Deafness caused by factors other than genetic abnormalities includes _____ and _____.

11. Pediatricians or ear, nose, and throat doctors (ENTs) insert _____ _____ in the ears of
    children who suffer from chronic _____ _____.

12. Almost all ear preparations contain several major ingredients such as _____ and _____.

MATCHING

Matching I
Match the following trade and generic drug names for eye prescriptions.

_____ 1. Trusopt
_____ 2. Xalatan
_____ 3. Voltaren
_____ 4. Decadron
_____ 5. Tobrex

A. Latanoprost
B. Dexamethasone
C. Tobramycin
D. Dorzolamide
E. Diclofenac

Matching II
Match the following medications or products with the ear conditions they treat.

_____ 1. Swim-Ear
_____ 2. Ciprodex
_____ 3. Cerumenex
_____ 4. Polymyxin B
_____ 5. Benzocaine

A. Ear tube infection
B. Pain associated with ear
   conditions
C. Bacterial external ear infections
D. Ear wax softening
E. Swimmer's ear

RESEARCH ACTIVITY

Follow the instructions given in each exercise and provide a response.

1. Visit a local pharmacy and locate the eye and ear care sections.
   A. What is the main ingredient in over-the-counter (OTC) eye drops?

   B. What is the main ingredient in OTC ear drops?

REFLECT CRITICALLY

CRITICAL THINKING

Reply to each question based on what you have learned in the chapter.

1. You have been working in the intravenous (IV) room all day, and your eyes are feeling very dry. What is the reason for your "dry eyes," and what can you do to resolve the situation?

2. Night blindness is often caused by a lack of vitamin A. What food can you eat to prevent night blindness?

3. Your child came home from school with "pinkeye." How can you prevent yourself from getting this contagious eye infection?

4. Why is sodium chloride (NaCl) an ingredient in every artificial tear product?

5. How is having an inner ear infection different from having a middle ear infection?

RELATE TO PRACTICE

LAB SCENARIOS

Therapeutic Agents for the Eyes, Ears, Nose, and Throat

Objective: To review with the pharmacy technician terms associated with the eyes, ears, nose, and throat and review the brand and generic name, indication, contraindications, adverse effects, dosage forms, routes of administration, and recommended daily dosage of medications used to treat disorders affecting the eyes, ears, nose and throat.

Lab Activity #19.1: Define the following terms associated with the eyes, ears, nose, and throat.

Equipment needed:

- Medical dictionary
- Pencil/pen

Time needed to complete this activity: 20 minutes.

1. Angle-closure glaucoma _____

2. Auralgia _____

3. Blepharitis _____

4. Conjunctivitis _____

5. Cysticercosis _____

6. Cytomegalovirus _____

7. Herpes simplex keratitis _____

8. Herpes zoster ophthalmicus _____

9. Iritis _____

10. Keratitis _____

11. Ocular toxoplasmosis _____

12. Open-angle glaucoma _____

13. Otalgia _____

14. Otitis externa _____

15. Otitis media _____

16. Otorrhea _____

17. Otosclerosis _____

18. Photopsia _____

19. Stye _____

20. Uveitis _____

21. Vertigo _____

Lab Activity #19.2: Using a drug reference book, identify the generic name, drug classification, indication, contraindications, adverse effects, dosage forms, routes of administration, and recommended daily dosage of medications used to treat conditions affecting the eyes, ears, nose, and throat.

Equipment needed:

- *Drug Facts & Comparisons* or *Physicians' Desk Reference*
- Pencil/pen

Time needed to complete this activity: 30 minutes

Brand (Trade) Name	Generic Name	Drug Classification	Indication	List Two Contraindications	List Five Adverse Effects	Dosage Forms Available	Routes of Administration	Recommended Daily Dosage
Alphagan P								
Antivert								
Cerumenex								
Ciloxan								
Ciprodex Otic								
Cortisporin Otic								
Cosopt								
Cytovene								
Foscavir								
Iopidine								
Lumigan								
Maxitrol								
Neosporin Ophthalmic								
Patanol								
Restasis								
Sulamyd								
Timoptic								
TobraDex								
Transderm Scop								
Travatan								
Trusopt								

TERMS AND DEFINITIONS

Select the correct term from the following list and write the corresponding letter in the blank next to the statement.

A. Analgesic
B. Antiinflammatory
C. Acne vulgaris
D. Antiseptic
E. Comedone
F. Dermis
G. Desquamation
H. Epidermis
I. Sebaceous glands
J. Keratolytic
K. Sebum
L. Skin protectant
M. Prophylaxis
N. Pruritus
O. Subcutaneous layer
P. Sweat glands
Q. Urticaria

___D___ 1. A substance that stops or slows the growth of microorganisms on surfaces such as skin

___K___ 2. Oily/waxy substance that lubricates the skin and keeps water in to provide moisture

___O___ 3. Deepest layer of skin that consists of fat cells and collagen

___A___ 4. Drug that relieves pain by reducing the perception of pain

___F___ 5. Thick layer of connective tissue that contains collagen

___N___ 6. Itching

___I___ 7. Skin glands responsible for secretion of an oily substance called sebum

___Q___ 8. Also known as hives; red welts that arise on the surface of the skin, often the result of an allergic reaction

___H___ 9. Outermost layer of the skin, composed of the stratum corneum or horny layer

___B___ 10. A drug that reduces swelling, redness, and pain and promotes healing

___L___ 11. A substance that acts as a barrier between the skin and any irritant

___C___ 12. Commonly known as pimples, this condition occurs when the pores of the skin are clogged with oil or bacteria

___J___ 13. A drug that causes shedding of the outer layer of the skin

___P___ 14. Found in the skin and used for cooling off the body when the temperature becomes too hot

___G___ 15. Process of shedding the top layer of the skin, also known as exfoliation

___M___ 16. Treatment given before a possible event to prevent the event from happening

___E___ 17. Blackhead; a plug of keratin and sebum within a hair follicle that is blackened at the surface

TRUE OR FALSE

Write T or F next to each statement.

___T___ 1. The skin is one of the most abused organs of the body system.

___F___ 2. The skin is one of the smallest organs in the body.

___F___ 3. The lunula is the small white portion at the tip of the nail.

___F___ 4. Growths on the surface of the skin are common and not all are cancerous.

___T___ 5. Therapy with blue light does not contain ultraviolet (UV) light that can damage the skin.

___F___ 6. Psoriasis is an uncommon and infectious inflammatory skin disorder.

___T___ 7. Burns range in severity from first degree to fourth degree; fourth degree is the most severe.

___F___ 8. Many canker sores will heal within a couple of months.

___T___ 9. Nails on both hands and feet endure daily abuse and can become damaged.

___T___10. Onychomycosis infection normally starts at the base of one or more toenails.

SYSTEM IDENTIFIER

Label the following parts of the skin.

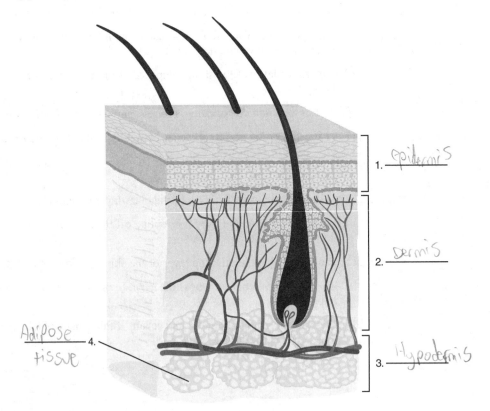

1. _Epidermis_

2. _Dermis_

3. _Hypodermis_

Adipose tissue — 4.

1. _____   3. _____

2. _____   4. _____

MULTIPLE CHOICE

Complete each question by circling the best answer.

1. The function of the skin is to protect the body against heat, cold, light, dehydration, and:
   A. Sunburn
   B. Injuries
   C. Infection
   D. Broken bones

2. The two glands that are within the layers of the skin are the sebaceous and _____ gland:
   A. Thyroid
   B. Sebum
   C. Sweat
   D. Lymph

3. Acne is a common condition caused by the inflammation of sebaceous glands that produce:
   A. Pustules
   B. Comedones
   C. Scars
   D. All of the above

4. Sunscreens protect the skin from:
   A. UVA rays
   B. Burning
   C. UVB rays
   D. A and C are correct

5. _____ are used to treat the symptoms of urticaria.
   A. Decongestants
   B. Antihistamines
   C. Sunscreens
   D. Ibuprofen

6. Abnormal growth of new tissue on the skin that results in a malignancy is known as:
   A. Skin cancer
   B. A skin tag
   C. A wart
   D. A nodule

7. Mild psoriasis covers _____ of the body.
   A. 3% to 10%
   B. 5% to 10%
   C. 10% to 20%
   D. 7% to 15%

8. A burn that penetrates the deepest layers of the skin, including muscles, tendons, and bones is:
   A. A third-degree burn
   B. A fourth-degree burn
   C. A second-degree burn
   D. A first-degree burn

9. Plantar warts are found on:
   A. The fingers around the knuckles
   B. The elbow
   C. The bottom of the foot
   D. The neck below the ears

10. Herpes zoster is caused by the varicella-zoster virus, which is the same virus that causes:
    A. Chickenpox
    B. Measles
    C. Mumps
    D. Pneumonia

11. Impetigo is highly contagious and the areas affected include:
    A. Abdomen
    B. Face
    C. Limbs
    D. All of the above

12. _____ _____ are caused by the parasite *Pediculus humanus capitis*.
    A. Cradle cap
    B. Head lice
    C. Athlete's foot
    D. Tapeworms

FILL IN THE BLANK

Answer each question by completing the statement in the space provided.

1. The nerves allow the skin to detect _____, _____, and _____.

2. Hair is made of proteins called _____ and is similar to the top layer of the skin.

3. The most effective non–drug treatment for acne is to _____

   _____.

4. UVA radiation is the longest _____ and makes up _____ of UV light.

5. The Skin Cancer Foundation recommends that people should avoid _____

   _____ and _____ _____.

6. Applying a _____ _____ _____ helps to alleviate the itching
   that accompanies hives.

7. _____ _____ _____ grows very slowly, occurs on the surface

of the skin, and is usually due to _____ _____.

8. Check your skin on a regular basis using the _____

_____.

9. _____ _____ is a condition caused by the build-up of fluids under the skin that
can cause ulcers.

10. Athlete's foot is caused by a fungus of the species _____ _____.

MATCHING

Match the term in the left column with the alternative name in the right column.

___C___ 1. Urticaria

___D___ 2. Genital warts

___E___ 3. Tinea pedis

___B___ 4. Canker sores

___A___ 5. Cold sores

A. Herpes simplex virus infection
B. Small topical ulcers
C. Hives
D. Human papillomavirus (HPV)
E. Athlete's foot

RESEARCH ACTIVITY

Follow the instructions given in each exercise and provide a response.

1. Access the website *http://www.fda.gov/Drugs/default.htm*. Locate Drugs@FDA and type in OTC (over the counter). Investigate and list what legend drugs have been converted to OTC status.

2. Access the website *http://www.cdc.gov/std/hpv/stdfact-hpv.htm*.
   A. How does HPV cause genital warts and cancer?

   B. Research information about the HPV vaccine Gardasil.

CRITICAL THINKING

Reply to each question based on what you have learned in the chapter.

1. Jamie is a pharmacy technician in a local retail store. A patient is complaining that her skin condition is worsening while using the prescribed antibacterial agent. Jamie directs the patient to the pharmacist for counseling. What will the pharmacist most likely tell the patient?

   She is probably having an allergic reaction to the antibacterial agent, or it may not be antibac bacteria-caused (her skin cond'n)

2. A patient is prescribed a corticosteroid ointment for psoriasis. Describe some of the possible side effects, especially if used long term.

   Side effects include skin redness, burning, itching, blistering of skin, crusting of treated skin.

3. Cathy goes to the doctor shortly after giving birth and returning home from the hospital. She is complaining of vaginal itching. On further questioning, she reveals that her newborn has "white spots" in her mouth. What do you suspect may be the problem, and what might be prescribed?

   Did Cathy have genital herpes and passed it to her newborn? Or maybe she passed HPV though no warts are present. The infant may have conker sores, and Cathy may have some kind of tinea cruris jock itch. Antifungal cream is the way.

4. Gus is a pharmacy technician in a specialty hospital. A patient is brought in with multiple severe burns. What special precautions would Gus need to observe when preparing medication for this patient?

   must be sterile, apply w/ sterile gloves

LAB SCENARIOS

Therapeutic Agents for the Integumentary System

Objective: To review with the pharmacy technician terms associated with the integumentary system and review the brand and generic names, indication, contraindications, adverse effects, dosage forms, routes of administration, and daily dosage of medications used to treat disorders of the integumentary system.

Lab Activity #20.1: Define the following terms associated with the integumentary system.

Equipment needed:

- Medical dictionary
- Pencil/pen

Time needed to complete this activity: 30 minutes.

1. Acne _____

2. Acne vulgaris _____

3. Allergy _____

4. Blister _____

5. Candidiasis _____

6. Comedone _____

7. Cysts _____

8. Decubitus ulcer _____

9. Dermatitis _____

10. Eczema _____

11. Fungus _____

12. Mycoses _____

13. Onychomycosis _____

14. Papule _____

15. Psoriasis _____

16. Pustule _____

17. Ringworm _____

18. Scabies _____

19. Tinea capitis _____

20. Tinea manus _____

21. Tinea pedis _____

22. Tinea unguium _____

23. Urticaria _____

24. Wheal _____

Lab Activity #20.2: Using a drug reference book, identify the generic name, drug classification, indication, contraindications, adverse effects, dosage forms, routes of administration, and daily dosage of medications used to treat conditions affecting the integumentary system.

Equipment needed:

- *Drug Facts & Comparisons* or *Physicians' Desk Reference*
- Pencil/pen

Time needed to complete this activity: 45 minutes

Brand (Trade) Name	Generic Name	Drug Classification	Indication	List Two Contraindications	List Five Adverse Effects	Dosage Forms Available	Routes of Administration	Recommended Daily Dosage
Accutane								
Aclovate								
AndroGel								
Azelex								
Bactroban								
Benzac								
BenzaClin								
Clobex								
Differin								
Diflucan								
Dovonex								
Dynacin								
Gris-Peg								
Lamisil								
Lidoderm								
Loprox								

Chapter **20 Integumentary System**

MetroCream	MetroGel	Minocin	Nizoral	Renagel	Renova	Retin-A	Silvadene	Spectazole	Sporanox	Sumycin	Tazorac	Terazol 7	Topicort	Ultravate	Vibramycin	Westcort

279

TERMS AND DEFINITIONS

Select the correct term from the following list and write the corresponding letter in the blank next to the statement.

A. Absorption
B. Amino acids
C. Appendicitis
D. Carbohydrates
E. Chyme
F. Constipation
G. Diarrhea
H. Digestion
I. Emesis
J. Excretion
K. Gastritis
L. Peptic ulcer
M. Ingestion
N. Lipids
O. Peristalsis
P. Ulcer
Q. Villus

_____ 1. Inflammation of the appendix

_____ 2. Fats and fatty acids

_____ 3. Frequent, watery, and loose stools

_____ 4. Inflammation of the stomach lining

_____ 5. A lesion on a mucous surface of the gastrointestinal (GI) tract

_____ 6. Molecules that make up proteins

_____ 7. An ulcerative condition of the lower esophagus, stomach, or duodenum usually caused by the bacterium *Helicobacter pylori*

_____ 8. Vomiting

_____ 9. The movement of nutrients, fluids, and medications from the GI tract into the bloodstream.

_____10. The soupy consistency of food after it has mixed with stomach acids and as it passes into the small intestine

_____11. Chemical substances made up of only carbon, hydrogen, and oxygen (e.g., sugars, starches, and cellulose)

_____12. To take in food or liquid

_____13. A projection from the surface of a mucous membrane

_____14. Elimination of waste products through stools and urine

_____15. The mechanical, chemical, and enzymatic action of breaking down food into molecules that can be used in metabolism

_____16. The contraction and relaxation of the tubular molecules of the esophagus, stomach, and intestines that move food from the mouth to the anus

_____17. The presence of dry, hard stools that may be decreased in frequency

TRUE OR FALSE

Write T or F next to each statement.

_____ 1. All medications used to treat symptoms of the digestive tract and intestines are prescription only.

_____ 2. The GI system is controlled by the sympathetic system.

_____ 3. The pharynx connects the mouth to the esophagus.

_____ 4. The small intestine is about 6 feet in length.

_____ 5. The small intestine is connected to the liver and the pancreas.

_____ 6. The gallbladder aids digestion by releasing bile.

_____ 7. The colon is the shortest section of the intestinal tract.

_____ 8. The appendix plays a vital role in the digestive system.

_____ 9. The mouth comes in contact with many kinds of bacteria every day.

_____10. Some proton pump inhibitors and H_2-antagonists are available in lesser strengths over the counter (OTC).

SYSTEM IDENTIFIER

Identify each organ/anatomical part in this system and enter the term next to the corresponding number.

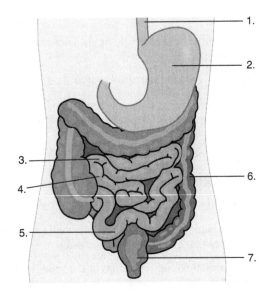

1. _____   5. _____

2. _____   6. _____

3. _____   7. _____

4. _____

MULTIPLE CHOICE

Complete each question by circling the best answer.

1. Which of the following is ***not*** a main function of the GI system?
   A. Digestion
   B. Absorption
   C. Metabolism
   D. Production of flatus

2. Which of the following is ***not*** a salivary gland?
   A. Subcutaneous
   B. Sublingual
   C. Submandibular
   D. Parotid

3. The function of the epiglottis is to close off the _____ so that food does not enter the wrong tube.
   A. Pharynx
   B. Trachea
   C. Esophagus
   D. Colon

4. Most absorption takes place in the:
   A. Duodenum
   B. Jejunum
   C. Ileum
   D. All of the above

5. What are the main sections of the large intestines?
   A. Cecum and ileum
   B. Rectum and jejunum
   C. Colon and rectum
   D. A and B

6. Which of the following is ***not*** a common condition that affects the GI system?
   A. Heartburn
   B. Appendicitis
   C. Constipation
   D. Diarrhea

7. The abbreviated term *s/s* means:
   A. Swish and swallow
   B. Sit and spin
   C. Swish and spit
   D. A and C

8. Simethicone is indicated for:
   A. Flatulence
   B. Diarrhea
   C. Heartburn
   D. Constipation

9. Aluminum can cause:
   A. Flatulence
   B. Diarrhea
   C. Heartburn
   D. Constipation

10. If a patient is vomiting, the physician may prescribe:
    A. Axid
    B. Colace
    C. Compazine
    D. Lomotil

FILL IN THE BLANK

Answer each question by completing the statement in the space provided.

1. The act of building molecules is known as _____, and the act of breaking down molecules to release energy is called _____.

2. The environment of the stomach is a more _____ pH, and the environment of the intestines is a more _____ pH.

3. Lack of good _____ hygiene is the most common reason conditions affecting the mouth occur.

4. Symptoms of throat inflammation include _____ _____ and _____.

5. Common dosage forms used in the oral cavity include _____, _____, _____, and _____.

6. High acid content of stomach fluids commonly contributes to _____, _____, _____, or _____.

7. _____ _____ _____ are used primarily in the treatment of GERD and peptic ulcer.

8. *H. pylori* is treated with a combination of _____ and _____ _____ medications.

9. _____ are common causes of diarrhea or constipation, along with other GI side effects.

10. Kaopectate, Fibercon, and Pepto-Bismol, used to treat diarrhea, are available _____.

11. _____ _____ _____ is a common condition marked by chronic or periodic diarrhea or constipation.

12. A common side effect of chemotherapy is _____.

MATCHING

Matching I
Match the following trade and generic drug names.

_____ 1. Pepcid

_____ 2. Prevacid

_____ 3. Dulcolax

_____ 4. Imodium

_____ 5. Compazine

A. Bisacodyl
B. Loperamide
C. Famotidine
D. Prochlorperazine
E. Lansoprazole

Matching II
Match the following drug classes with the correct example.

_____ 1. Tagamet

_____ 2. Prilosec

_____ 3. Fibercon

_____ 4. Reglan

_____ 5. Ipecac

A. Antidiarrheal
B. Antiemetic
C. H2-antagonist
D. Emetic
E. Proton pump inhibitor

SHORT ANSWER

Write a short response to each question in the space provided.

1. What is the sequence of organs in the GI tract?

_____

_____

_____

2. What is the important function of the intrinsic factor found in the stomach?

_____

_____

_____

3. As of April 2008, the Food and Drug Administration (FDA) required new labeling on Ipecac stating:

_____

_____

_____

RESEARCH ACTIVITY

Follow the instructions given in each exercise and provide a response.

1. Many prescription medications for GI upset and heartburn have been changed to OTC status. Visit the website *www.fda.gov* and make a list of the GI medications that are now available OTC and the difference in dosage strengths compared with when these drugs were prescription medications.

2. Visit the website *www.cvs.com*. Compare prices of the medications you listed in question 1.

REFLECT CRITICALLY

CRITICAL THINKING

Reply to each question based on what you have learned in the chapter.

1. It has been stated that you must chew your food "32 times." How does not chewing your food affect digestion in the stomach?

2. A hectic and stressful lifestyle can contribute to many "stomach problems" such as indigestion and acid-reflux. What lifestyle changes can be made to reduce these problems?

3. What constitutes good oral hygiene? Is flossing that important?

4. Many articles recommend drinking eight glasses of water a day. What are some of the benefits of doing so?

5. Is bulimia a psychological or a physical condition?

RELATE TO PRACTICE

LAB SCENARIOS

Therapeutic Agents for the Gastrointestinal System

Objective: To review with the pharmacy technician terms associated with the GI system and review the brand and generic names, indication, contraindications, adverse effects, dosage forms, routes of administration, and recommended daily dosage of medications used to treat disorders of the endocrine system.

Lab Activity #21.1: Define the following terms associated with the GI system.

DID YOU KNOW?
- 29.3 million (8.6%) adults are diagnosed with ulcers.
- 35.9 million visits to office-based physicians with diseases of the digestive system as the primary diagnosis.
- 67% of adults age 20 years and older are overweight or obese.

Equipment needed:

- Medical dictionary
- Pencil/pen

Time needed to complete this activity: 15 minutes.

1. Appendicitis _____

2. Constipation _____

3. Diarrhea _____

4. Duodenal ulcer _____

5. Crohn's disease _____

287

6. Fistula _____

7. Gastric ulcer _____

8. Gastroesophageal reflux disease (GERD) _____

9. Hiatal hernia _____

10. Inflammatory bowel syndrome (IBS) _____

11. Irritable bowel disease (IBD) _____

12. Laryngopharyngeal reflux _____

13. Peptic ulcer disease (PUD) _____

14. Reflux _____

15. Ulcerative colitis _____

Lab Activity #21.2: Using a drug reference book, identify the generic name, drug classification, indication, contraindications, adverse effects, dosage forms, routes of administration, and recommended daily dosage of medications used to treat conditions affecting the GI system.

Equipment Needed:

- *Drug Facts & Comparisons or Physicians' Desk Reference*
- Pencil/pen

Time needed to complete this activity: 30 minutes

Brand (Trade) Name	Generic Name	Drug Classification	Indication	List Two Contraindications	List Five Adverse Effects	Dosage Forms Available	Routes of Administration	Recommended Daily Dosage
AcipHex								
Asacol								
Axid								
Azulfidine								
Bentyl								
Cytotec								
Dipentum								
Imuran								
Lomotil								
Nexium								
Pentasa								
Pepcid								
Prevacid								
Prevpac								
Protonix								
Reglan								
Tagamet								
Zantac								

22 Urinary System

REINFORCE KEY CONCEPTS

TERMS AND DEFINITIONS

Select the correct term from the following list and write the corresponding letter in the blank next to the statement.

A. Acidification
B. Acidosis
C. Alkalosis
D. Blood urea nitrogen
E. Dialysis
F. Distribution
G. Diuretic
H. Electrolyte
I. Excretion
J. Kidney stones
K. Micturition
L. Nephrons
M. Osmosis
N. Renal absorption
O. Renal artery
P. Renal failure
Q. Renal fascia
R. Renal metabolism
S. Renal vein
T. Tubular reabsorption
U. Tubular secretion
V. Urea
W. Ureter
X. Urethra

_____ 1. Inability of the kidneys to function properly

_____ 2. Charged elements called cations and anions; key elements are sodium and potassium

_____ 3. Test that measures the nitrogen in the blood in the form of urea

_____ 4. Filtering unit of the kidneys

_____ 5. Agent that increases urine output and excretion of water from the body

_____ 6. One of the pair of arteries that branch off from the abdominal aorta

_____ 7. Tube by which filtered blood from the kidneys is sent back into the body's circulatory system

_____ 8. Urination

_____ 9. Passage of a solute through a semipermeable membrane to remove toxic materials/wastes and to maintain fluid, electrolyte, and pH levels of the body system

_____10. Conversion to an acidic environment

_____11. Within the kidneys; the mechanism by which elements are sent throughout the body

_____12. Diffusion of water from low solute concentrations to higher solute concentrations

_____13. Increase of alkalinity of the blood resulting from the accumulation of alkali or reduction of acid content

_____14. Membranous tissue that surrounds and supports the kidneys

_____15. Elimination of waste products through stools and urine

_____16. Within the kidneys; mechanism by which chemical transformation takes place

_____17. Conservation of protein, glucose, bicarbonate, and water from the glomerular filtrated by the tubules

_____18. Within the kidneys; the intake of liquids, solids, and gases

_____19. Increase of acid content of the blood resulting from the accumulation of acid or loss of bicarbonate

_____20. Solid mineral deposits that form in the urinary tract

_____21. Tube that carries urine from the bladder to the outside where it is eliminated

_____22. Function of the nephron in which ions, toxins, and water are secreted into the collecting duct to be excreted

_____23. Tube that carries urine from the kidneys to the bladder

_____24. Main nitrogenous constituent of urine and final product of protein metabolism

291

TRUE OR FALSE

Write T or F next to each statement.

_____ 1. The shape of the kidneys is similar to the shape of a kidney bean.

_____ 2. When the kidney is full, the person feels the need to urinate.

_____ 3. The body excretes about 960 ml of urine per day.

_____ 4. Each kidney contains millions of microscopic nephrons.

_____ 5. The ureters lead to the bladder.

_____ 6. It is impossible for people to survive without two functioning kidneys.

_____ 7. Drinking plenty of water is one of the most effective ways to take care of the urinary system.

_____ 8. Younger adults suffer from acute renal failure more often then older people.

_____ 9. Men are more susceptible to urinary tract infections (UTIs) than are women.

_____10. Incontinence tends to affect women more than men.

SYSTEM IDENTIFIER

Identify each main organ/anatomical part in the urinary system and enter the term next to the corresponding number.

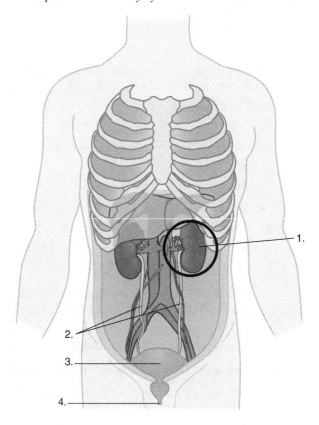

1. _____   3. _____

2. _____   4. _____

Label the parts of the kidney.

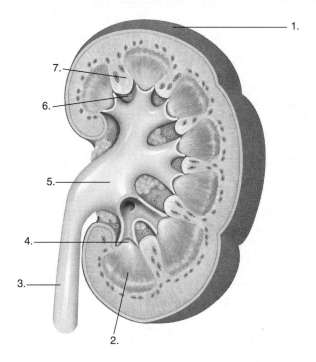

1. _____   5. _____

2. _____   6. _____

3. _____   7. _____

4. _____

MULTIPLE CHOICE

Complete each question by circling the best answer.

1. The urge to urinate is called:
   A. Maturation
   B. Micturition
   C. Acidification
   D. Excretion

2. What volume of blood products do the kidneys filter each day?
   A. 0.5 gallons
   B. 5 gallons
   C. 50 gallons
   D. 500 gallons

3. Albumins and globulins are components of:
   A. Plasma
   B. Blood
   C. Hemoglobin
   D. All of the above

4. The one-way reabsorption of sodium and chloride from the loop of Henle is called:
   A. Ion exchange
   B. Osmosis
   C. Active transport
   D. Tubular secretion

5. The productions of a large volume of urine within a certain period of time is called:
   A. Anuria
   B. Oliguria
   C. Polyuria
   D. Uremia

6. Which of the following is a symptom of end-stage renal disease (ESRD)?
   A. Congestive heart failure (CHF)
   B. Pulmonary edema
   C. Nausea and vomiting
   D. All of the above

7. A nosocomial infection is an infection:
   A. Of the nose
   B. Acquired in the hospital or health care setting
   C. Acquired while in a coma
   D. None of the above

8. Which of the following is *not* a means of cleansing the blood of patients with ESRD?
   A. Hemodialysis
   B. Peritoneal dialysis
   C. Nocturnal dialysis
   D. Oxydialysis

9. The most common side effect of all thiazide-like agents is:
   A. Frequent urination
   B. Infrequent urination
   C. Increased thiamine levels
   D. Decreased thiamine levels

10. Kegel exercises are done to help overcome:
    A. Stress
    B. Incontinence
    C. CHF
    D. UTIs

FILL IN THE BLANK

Answer each question by completing the statement in the space provided.

1. The four major functions of the body are _____, _____, _____, and _____.

2. _____ occurs when too many free hydrogen ions are present, and _____ occurs when too many hydroxide ions are present.

3. The portion of the kidneys that actually does the work of separation is the _____.

4. Two important functions of the nephron are _____ _____ and _____ _____.

5. The acid content in urine is between a pH of _____ and _____.

6. An example of a buffer is _____.

7. Two types of edema are _____ and _____.

8. One of the most common conditions affecting the urinary system is _____.

9. People receiving dialysis must watch their _____ and _____ intake.

10. The mechanism of action for thiazides and thiazide-like agents is that they equally _____ the urinary excretion of the ions _____ and _____.

MATCHING

Matching I

Match the following medical terms with their definitions.

_____ 1. Anuria

_____ 2. Cystitis

_____ 3. Urethritis

_____ 4. Hypokalemia

_____ 5. Pyelonephritis

A. Inflammation of the urethra
B. Inflammation of the kidney
C. Excessive decrease in potassium in the blood
D. Lack of urine
E. Inflammation of the bladder

Matching II

Match the following trade names with their generic drug names.

_____ 1. Diuril

_____ 2. Lasix

_____ 3. Aldactone

_____ 4. Diamox

_____ 5. Macrodantin

A. Spironolactone
B. Acetazolamide
C. Chlorothiazide
D. Nitrofurantoin
E. Furosemide

295

Write a short response to each question in the space provided.

1. Name the six main classes of diuretics used to treat edema.

   _____

   _____

   _____

   _____

   _____

2. What are the symptoms of a kidney stone?

   _____

   _____

   _____

3. Who is at high risk for renal failure?

   _____

   _____

   _____

RESEARCH ACTIVITY

Follow the instructions given in each exercise and provide a response.

1. Visit the website *www.healthandage.com*. Investigate and list the benefits of cranberries for the treatment of UTIs.

2. Visit the website *www.yoga-for-health-and-fitness.com*. Investigate and list the benefits of drinking eight glasses of water a day.

3. Research dialysis treatment, and list the process.

CRITICAL THINKING

Reply to each question based on what you have learned in the chapter.

1. Methicillin-resistant *Staphylococcus aureus* (MRSA) is a well-known nosocomial infection. Patients in the intensive care unit are quite susceptible to MRSA. What are some ways to prevent the spread of this type of infection?

2. If a UTI is left untreated, how will the infection progress?

3. Diabetes can be complicated by hypertension and kidney failure. A change in the patient's diet is always recommended. Apply your knowledge of the disease and devise a list of lifestyle changes that would benefit a diabetic patient.

RELATE TO PRACTICE

LAB SCENARIOS

Therapeutic Agents for the Urinary System
Objective: To review with the pharmacy technician the organs of the urinary system.

> **DID YOU KNOW?**
> - 3.7 million (1.7%) adults are diagnosed with kidney disease.
> - Kidney disease is the ninth leading cause of death.

Lab Activity #22.1: Define the following terms associated with the urinary system.

Equipment needed:

- Medical dictionary
- Pencil/pen

Time needed to complete this activity: 15 minutes

1. Benign prostatic hyperplasia (BPH) _____

2. Dehydration _____

3. Edema _____

4. Hyperchloremia _____

297

5. Hyperkalemia _____

6. Hypernatremia _____

7. Hyperphosphatemia _____

8. Hypocalcemia _____

9. Hypochloremia _____

10. Hypokalemia _____

11. Hyponatremia _____

12. Hypophosphatemia _____

13. Incontinence _____

14. Prostate disease _____

Lab Activity #22.2: Using a drug reference book, identify the generic name, drug classification, indications, contraindications, adverse effects, dosage forms, routes of administration, and recommended daily dosage of medications used to treat conditions affecting the renal system.

Equipment needed:

- *Drug Facts & Comparisons or Physicians' Desk Reference*
- Pencil/pen

Time needed to complete this activity: 15 minutes.

Brand (Trade) Name	Generic Name	Drug Classification	Indication	List Two Contraindications	List Five Adverse Effects	Dosage Forms Available	Routes of Administration	Recommended Daily Dosage
Avodart								
Bumex								
Cardura								
Caverject								
Cialis								
Flomax								
Hytrin								
Klor-Con								
Lasix								
Levitra								
Proscar								
Uroxatral								
Viagra								

23 Cardiovascular System

TERMS AND DEFINITIONS

Select the correct term from the following list and write the corresponding letter in the blank next to the statement.

A. Vena cava
B. Artery
C. Capillary
D. Coagulation
E. Diuretic
F. Endocardium
G. Enzyme
H. Thrombin
I. Thrombolytic
J. Vein
K. Syndrome
L. Pericardium
M. Embolism
N. Epicardium
O. Myocardium

_____ 1. Medication used to break up a thrombus or blood clot

_____ 2. A vessel that carries oxygenated blood from the heart to the tissues of the body

_____ 3. Thin membrane that lines the interior of the heart

_____ 4. An agent that increases urine output and excretion of water from the body

_____ 5. A vessel that carries deoxygenated blood to the heart

_____ 6. To solidify or change from a fluid state to a solid state as in forming a blood clot

_____ 7. Protein that speeds up a reaction by reducing the amount of energy required to initiate a reaction

_____ 8. Large veins that bring deoxygenated blood from the upper and lower part of the body to the right atrium of the heart

_____ 9. An enzyme formed in coagulating blood that forms blood clots

_____10. Extremely small vessel that connects the ends of the smallest arteries to the smallest veins and where the exchange of nutrients and waste, oxygen, and carbon dioxide occurs

_____11. Set of conditions

_____12. Muscle tissue layer of the heart

_____13. Formation of a clot from any substance that obstructs a vessel

_____14. Fluid-filled membrane that surrounds the heart

_____15. Inner layer of the pericardium

TRUE OR FALSE

Write T or F next to each statement.

_____ 1. A normal heart beats 160 to 200 times per minute.

_____ 2. The right atrium receives oxygenated blood from the lungs and pumps it out to the body.

_____ 3. The cardiac conduction system provides the electrical charge that makes the heart pump.

_____ 4. Most of the body's blood supply is cycled through the heart in 1 minute.

_____ 5. Congestive heart failure (CHF) is a condition in which the heart cannot pump as vigorously as necessary to deliver blood throughout the body.

_____ 6. The good cholesterol is known as *LDL*.

_____ 7. High blood pressure is also known as the "silent killer" because it has no obvious signs.

_____ 8. Sublingual nitroglycerin is good for only 6 months after the container is opened.

_____ 9. A person suffering from hypotension has high blood pressure.

_____10. Diet and exercise can lower lipid content.

Identify each component in the heart system and enter the term next to the corresponding number.

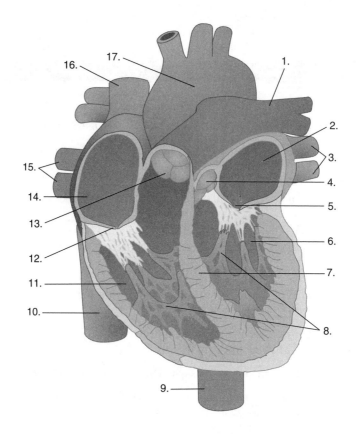

1. _____

2. _____

3. _____

4. _____

5. _____

6. _____

7. _____

8. _____

9. _____

10. _____

11. _____

12. _____

13. _____

14. _____

15. _____

16. _____

17. _____

MULTIPLE CHOICE

Complete each question by circling the best answer.

1. Tenormin, Inderal, and Lopressor are all classified as:
   A. Angiotensin-converting enzyme (ACE) inhibitors
   B. Beta blockers
   C. Calcium channel blockers
   D. Diuretics

2. Which of the following is ***not*** a main layer of the heart?
   A. Endocardium
   B. Myocardium
   C. Subcardium
   D. Epicardium

3. Pain and pressure in the chest caused by a lack of blood flow and oxygenation of the heart muscle are primary features of:
   A. Angina pectoris
   B. Arrhythmia
   C. Hyperlipidemia
   D. High blood pressure

4. Which of the following is ***not*** a greater risk factor for hypertension?
   A. Age
   B. Gender
   C. Race
   D. None of the above

5. An *embolus* is a:
   A. Blood clot
   B. Hemorrhage
   C. Rise in blood pressure
   D. Rise in lipid levels

6. Lovastatin, simvastatin, and pravastatin are classified as:
   A. Antihypertensives
   B. Antiarrhythmics
   C. Anticoagulants
   D. Antihyperlipidemics

7. A code blue situation can occur when a patient:
   A. Is having a heart attack
   B. Quits breathing
   C. A and B
   D. None of the above

8. An antidote for an overdose of Lanoxin is:
   A. Digoxin
   B. Digibind
   C. Digitalis
   D. Digitonin

9. Which of the following is *not* an element of the four-step approach to controlling high blood pressure?
   A. Weight reduction
   B. Diuretics
   C. Antianginals
   D. Beta blockers

10. Nitrostat tablets should be administered by which route?
    A. PO
    B. SL
    C. SubQ
    D. PR

FILL IN THE BLANK

Answer each question by completing the statement in the space provided.

1. The main arteries that supply blood to the heart are called _____ _____.

2. _____ is a syndrome that affects arterial blood vessels.

3. A thrombus in the heart can cause a _____ _____.

4. Cholesterol is important for the making of _____ _____ and

   _____ _____.

5. A cholesterol level below _____ indicates overall low cholesterol.

6. A category of drugs available over the counter (OTC) that can increase blood pressure are the

   _____.

7. Nitrates are used in the treatment of _____.

8. If plaque increases to form a blood clot, a _____ is created. This eventually may close off the
   vessel, causing a _____.

9. _____ and _____ are two side effects of hypotension.

10. Niacin, including forms available OTC, can lower _____.

MATCHING

Match the classes of drugs.

_____ 1. Antihyperlipidemics

_____ 2. Arrhythmic agents

_____ 3. Cardioglycosides

_____ 4. Antihypertensives

_____ 5. Anticoagulants

A. Quinidine, procainamide, verapamil
B. Heparin, warfarin
C. ACE inhibitors, beta blockers, calcium channel blockers
D. Bile acid sequestrants, HMG-CoA reductase inhibitors
E. Digoxin

DRUG NAMES

Give the generic names for the following drugs.

1. Mevacor _____

2. Norpace _____

3. Lanoxin _____

4. Dyrenium _____

5. Lotensin _____

6. Hytrin _____

7. Quinidex _____

8. Zestril _____

9. Cozaar _____

10. Cardizem _____

SHORT ANSWER

Reply to each question based on what you have learned in the chapter.

1. How do ACE inhibitors help reduce blood pressure?

   _____

   _____

   _____

2. How do calcium channel blockers work?

   _____

   _____

   _____

RESEARCH ACTIVITY

Follow the instructions given in each exercise and provide a response.

1. Access the website *www.americanheart.org*. What is tPA? How does this drug help stroke victims recover?

2. Access the website *www.rxlist.com*. Locate Side Effects and Drug Interactions. What are the side effects of aspirin and with what drugs does it interact?

CRITICAL THINKING

Reply to each question based on what you have learned in the chapter.

1. "An aspirin a day keeps a heart attack away." What are some everyday activities people can do to "keep a heart attack away"?

2. You have just finished your lunch, which consisted of a double cheeseburger, extra large fries, and a cola. Name all the body systems that will be affected by that "yummy" meal.

3. When people are asked to change their lifestyle as a result of life-threatening diseases (such as after a myocardial infarction [MI]), what two words do they dread hearing?

4. "I feel like I'm having a heart attack," someone says to you. How do you know for sure? What symptoms do you look for?

LAB SCENARIOS

Therapeutic Agents for the Cardiovascular System

Objective: To review with the pharmacy technician terms associated with the cardiovascular system and review the brand and generic names, indication, contraindications, adverse effects, dosage forms, routes of administration, and recommended daily dosage of medications used to treat disorders of the cardiovascular system.

DID YOU KNOW?

- In 2006, 631,636 people died of heart disease. Heart disease caused 26% of all deaths.
- Heart disease is ranked as the leading cause of death.
- Heart disease is the leading cause of death for both men and women. Half of the deaths caused by heart disease were in women.
- Coronary heart disease is the most common type of heart disease.
- Every year about 785,000 Americans have a first heart attack. Another 470,000 who have already had one or more heart attacks have another attack.
- In 2010, heart disease will cost the United States $316.4 billion. This total includes the cost of health care services, medications, and lost productivity.
- 25.8% of all deaths in African Americans is attributed to heart disease.
- 32% of all adults age 20 and older are diagnosed with hypertension.
- 16% of all adults age 20 years and older suffer from high serum cholesterol.
- 7.1 % of visits to office-based physicians result in cholesterol being measured.
- 6.5 million (2.9%) of adults have been diagnosed with a stroke.

Lab Activity #23.1: Define the following terms associated with the cardiovascular system.

Equipment needed:

- Medical dictionary
- Pencil/pen

Time needed to complete this activity: 30 minutes.

1. Aneurysm _____

2. Angina _____

3. Anoxia _____

4. Aorta _____

5. Arrhythmia _____

6. Arteriosclerosis _____

7. Atherosclerosis _____

8. Atrial fibrillation _____

9. Atrial flutter _____

10. Bradycardia _____

11. Cardiomyopathy _____

12. CHF _____

13. Deep vein thrombosis (DVT) _____

14. Diastolic blood pressure _____

15. Embolic stroke _____

16. Endocarditis _____

17. Heart failure _____

18. Hemorrhagic stroke _____

19. Hyperkalemia _____

20. Hyperlipidemia _____

21. Hypernatremia _____

22. Hypertension _____

23. Hypokalemia _____

24. Hyponatremia _____

25. Hypotension _____

26. Hypoxia _____

27. Infarction _____

28. Ischemia _____

29. Mitral valve prolapse _____

30. Mitral valve stenosis _____

31. MI _____

32. Orthostatic hypotension _____

33. Peripheral vascular disease _____

34. Phlebitis _____

35. Plaque _____

36. Prehypertension _____

37. Raynaud disease _____

38. Rheumatic heart disease _____

39. Stable angina _____

40. Stroke _____

41. Supraventricular tachycardia _____

42. Systolic blood pressure _____

43. Tachycardia _____

44. Thrombophlebitis _____

45. Thrombosis _____

46. Thrombotic stroke _____

47. Thrombus _____

48. Transient ischemic attack (TIA) _____

49. Unstable angina _____

50. Variant angina _____

51. Ventricular fibrillation _____

52. Ventricular tachycardia _____

Lab Activity #23.2: Using a drug reference book, identify the generic name, drug classification, indication, contraindications, adverse effects, dosage forms, routes of administration, and recommended daily dosage of medications used to treat conditions affecting the cardiovascular system.

Equipment needed:

- *Drug Facts & Comparisons* or *Physicians' Desk Reference*
- Pencil/pen

Time needed to complete the exercise: 60 minutes.

Brand (Trade) Name	Generic Name	Drug Classification	Indication	List Two Contraindications	List Five Adverse Effects	Dosage Forms Available	Routes of Administration	Recommended Daily Dosage
Aggrenox								
Aldactone								
Altace								
Atacand								
Avapro								
Benicar								
Benicar HCT								
Bumex								
Caduet								
Calan								
Cardizem								
Cardura								
Catapres-TTS								
Cordarone								
Coreg CR								
Coumadin								
Covera								
Cozaar								

Diovan						
Diovan HCT						
Dyazide						
Hytrin						
Hyzaar						
Imdur						
Inderal						
Isoptin						
Isordil						
Jantoven						
Klor-Con						
Lanoxin						
Lasix						
Lipitor						
Lovenox						
Lovenox						
Lozol						
Maxzide						
Mevacor						
Micardis						
Micardis HCT						

Continued

311

Brand (Trade) Name	Generic Name	Drug Classification	Indication	List Two Contraindications	List Five Adverse Effects	Dosage Forms Available	Routes of Administration	Recommended Daily Dosage
Niaspan								
Nitrostat								
Norpace								
Norvasc								
Plavix								
Prinivil								
Procardia								
Sectral								
Tambocor								
Tenormin								
Toprol XL								
TriCor								
Vasotec								
Verelan								
Vytorin								
WelChol								
Zestril								
Zetia								
Zocor								

24 Reproductive System

TERMS AND DEFINITIONS

Select the correct term from the following list and write the corresponding letter in the blank next to the statement.

A. Sperm
B. Endometrium
C. Fallopian tubes
D. Fertilization
E. Gametes
F. Inert ingredient
G. Menopause
H. Negative feedback
I. Oocyte or ova
J. Palliative
K. Teratogen
L. Abortifacients
M. Androgens
N. Chloasma
O. Depot

_____ 1. Brings relief but does not cure

_____ 2. Mucous membrane lining of the uterus

_____ 3. The female reproductive germ cell

_____ 4. An ingredient that has little or no effect on body functions

_____ 5. The narrow passages between the ovaries and the uterus

_____ 6. Any agent causing abnormal embryonic or fetal development

_____ 7. Sex cells, or ova and sperm

_____ 8. The process by which a sperm unites with an ovum to create a new life

_____ 9. A self-regulating mechanism in which the output of a system has input or control over the process

_____10. The male reproductive germ cell

_____11. Cessation of menstruation; a natural phenomenon in which a woman passes from a reproductive state to a non-reproductive state

_____12. Any treatment that causes abortion of a fetus

_____13. Male hormones

_____14. Area of the body in which a substance can accumulate or be stored for later distribution

_____15. Hyperpigmentation of skin that is limited/confined to a certain area, usually on the face during pregnancy

TRUE OR FALSE

Write T or F next to each statement.

_____ 1. The reproductive system is not interdependent on other body systems.

_____ 2. The gonads provide characteristics of both males and females.

_____ 3. The male reproductive system is closely tied to the endocrine system.

_____ 4. Women produce ova every month.

_____ 5. The female uterus houses the fertilized ovum.

_____ 6. Mammary gland tissue is regulated by hormonal secretions.

_____ 7. The hypothalamus can distinguish between natural and synthetic hormones.

_____ 8. Natural testosterone used for medicinal purposes is obtained from the testes of horses.

_____ 9. Oral contraceptives provide protection from sexually transmitted diseases.

_____10. The morning-after pill is a high-dose oral contraceptive.

Male Reproductive System

Identify each component in this system and enter the term next to the corresponding number.

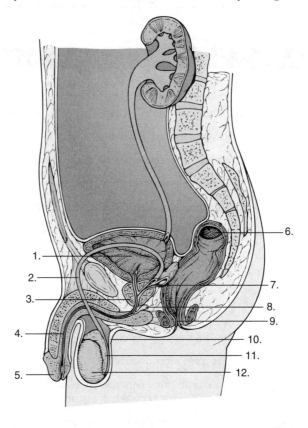

1. _____

2. _____

3. _____

4. _____

5. _____

6. _____

7. _____

8. _____

9. _____

10. _____

11. _____

12. _____

Female Reproductive System

Identify each component in this system and enter the term next to the corresponding number.

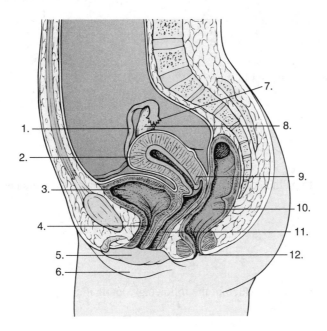

1. _____

2. _____

3. _____

4. _____

5. _____

6. _____

7. _____

8. _____

9. _____

10. _____

11. _____

12. _____

MULTIPLE CHOICE

Complete each question by circling the best answer.

1. The gonads or reproductive organs are responsible for:
   A. Secretion of hormones
   B. Production of sex cells
   C. Gender characteristics of males only
   D. A and B

2. Sperm production in males begins at puberty and continues until:
   A. Midlife
   B. Age 70
   C. Throughout the lifetime
   D. None of the above

3. The most abundant androgen is:
   A. Estrogen
   B. Testosterone
   C. Progesterone
   D. Inhibin

4. The ovum is most commonly fertilized in the:
   A. Uterus
   B. Cervix
   C. Ovary
   D. Fallopian tube

5. Female hormones are used to palliate conditions of the male reproductive tract such as:
   A. Prostate cancer
   B. Testicular cancer
   C. Impotence
   D. A and B

6. Oral contraceptives are formulated in which of the following combinations?
   A. Monophasic
   B. Biphasic
   C. Triphasic
   D. All of the above

7. The goal of treatment for benign prostatic hypertrophy is to:
   A. Relieve hesitancy of urination
   B. Decrease nocturia
   C. Prevent the development of urinary tract infections
   D. All of the above

8. Which of the following hormones is used to treat abnormal uterine bleeding, abnormal ovulation, and infertility?
   A. Progesterone
   B. Estrogen
   C. Testosterone
   D. Follicle-stimulating hormone

9. The source of conjugated estrogens used for hormone replacement therapy is:
   A. Plants
   B. Urine of pregnant mares
   C. Placentas
   D. A and B

10. Contraceptives given by injection prevent pregnancy by:
    A. Suppressing ovulation
    B. Thickening the cervical mucus
    C. Altering the endometrium
    D. All of the above

FILL IN THE BLANK

Answer each question by completing the statement in the space provided.

1. Patients taking _____ should not take sildenafil or related drugs for erectile dysfunction (ED) because the combination causes a dangerous decrease in blood pressure.

2. _____ is known as the abortion pill.

3. One cause of female infertility is _____.

4. The barrier types of contraceptives for females are _____, _____ _____, and _____.

5. Latex, polyurethane, and lamb intestine are three types of materials used to make _____.

6. Some of the serious risks of taking _____ _____ include thromboembolism, myocardial infarction, and stroke.

7. The side effects of _____ include weight gain, stomach pain, and stomach cramping.

8. _____ are one of the natural sources from which progestins can be obtained.

9. Oil-based injectable estrogen medications are called _____ medications.

10. Left untreated, some sexually transmitted diseases (STDs) can cause irreversible _____, _____, and even _____.

MATCHING

Matching I
Match the following trade and generic drug names.

_____ 1. Proscar

_____ 2. Flomax

_____ 3. Premarin

_____ 4. Ogen

_____ 5. Provera

A. Conjugated estrogens
B. Estropipate
C. Finasteride
D. Medroxyprogesterone
E. Tamsulosin

Matching II
Match the following trade and generic drug names.

_____ 1. Parlodel

_____ 2. Ortho Tri-Cyclen

_____ 3. Lo-Ovral

_____ 4. Hytrin

_____ 5. Viagra

A. Ethinyl estradiol/norgestrel
B. Sildenafil
C. Terazosin
D. Bromocriptine
E. Ethinyl estradiol/norgestimate

SHORT ANSWER

Write a short response to each question in the space provided.

1. Sildenafil (Viagra) was introduced in 1998 for the treatment of _____.

2. Any disease that can be transmitted by _____ _____ is considered an STD.

3. Androgens provide a sense of _____ _____, _____

   _____ and _____.

4. Combination oral contraceptives consist of both _____ and _____, which act to inhibit ovulation.

5. The primary actions of estrogens are to maintain reproductive structures such as _____

   _____ _____ and to provide _____

   _____ _____.

6. Androgens stimulate the formation of _____ _____ _____

   like increased _____ _____ and growth of _____

   _____.

RESEARCH ACTIVITY

Follow the instructions given in each exercise and provide a response.

1. Access the website *www.birthcontrol.com*. Research and list the latest developments in birth control for both males and females.

2. Access the website *www.niaid.nih.gov/factsheet/stdpid.htm*. Read about pelvic inflammatory disease and its effects on sexually active young women. Summarize what you have learned.

3. Access the website *http://webmd.lycos.com*. Type in "saw palmetto." Read the article, "An Herb for Prostate Problems?" Summarize what you have learned.

CRITICAL THINKING

Reply to each question based on what you have learned in the chapter.

1. Women have been told for many years that when menopause occurs, they will need hormonal replacement therapy (HRT). However, recently released information indicates that long-term HRT is more harmful than beneficial. What advice will you give women on this subject?

2. Birth control has been taught in middle schools and high schools for many years in an attempt to curb teen pregnancy. Why is the rate of teen pregnancy still high?

3. Propecia was approved by the Food and Drug Administration (FDA) for the treatment of hair loss. The active ingredient in Propecia is finasteride, which is the same drug used to treat benign prostatic hypertrophy, known by the brand name Proscar. What is the difference in strength between Propecia and Proscar, and what are the side effects of finasteride?

RELATE TO PRACTICE

LAB SCENARIOS

Therapeutic Agents for the Reproductive System

Objective: To review with the pharmacy technician terms associated with the organs of the reproductive system and review the brand and generic names, indication, contraindications, adverse effects, dosage forms, routes of administration, and recommended daily dosage of medications used to treat disorders of the reproductive system.

DID YOU KNOW?
- 19% of women aged 15 to 44 currently use oral contraceptives.
- 7.3 million (11.8%) women ages 15 to 44 have impaired ability to have children.
- In 2007, there were 1,108,374 new cases of chlamydia.

Lab Activity #24.1: Define the following terms associated with the reproductive system.

Equipment needed:

- Medical dictionary

- Pencil/pen

Time needed to complete this activity: 15 minutes.

1. Amenorrhea _____

2. Dysfunctional uterine bleeding (DUB) _____

3. Dysmenorrhea _____

4. Endometriosis _____

5. Erectile dysfunction _____

6. Hypogonadism _____

7. Infertility _____

8. Kallmann's syndrome _____

9. Klinefelter's syndrome _____

10. Menopause _____

11. Pelvic inflammatory disease (PID) _____

12. Pregnancy _____

13. Premenstrual syndrome (PMS) _____

14. Salpingitis _____

15. Vaginitis _____

Lab Activity #24.2: Using a drug reference book, identify the generic name, drug classification, indication, contraindications, adverse effects, dosage forms, routes of administration, and recommended daily dosage of medications used to treat conditions affecting the reproductive system.

Equipment needed:

- *Drug Facts & Comparisons* or *Physicians' Desk Reference*

- Pencil/pen

Time needed to complete this activity: 60 minutes.

Brand (Trade) Name	Generic Name	Drug Classification	Indication	List Two Contraindications	List Five Adverse Effects	Dosage Forms Available	Routes of Administration	Recommended Daily Dosage
Alesse								
Apiri								
Cialis								
Climara								
Clomid								
Danocrine								
Estrace								
Estraderm								
Femhrt								
Junel								
Levitra								
Loestrin 24 Fe								
Lupron								
NuvaRing								
Ortho Novum								
Ortho Tri-Cyclen								

Continued

321

Brand (Trade) Name	Generic Name	Drug Classification	Indication	List Two Contraindications	List Five Adverse Effects	Dosage Forms Available	Routes of Administration	Recommended Daily Dosage
Ortho-Cyclen								
Ortho Tri-Cyclen Lo								
Parlodel								
Pergonal								
Plan B								
Premarin								
Premphase								
Prempro								
Prempro								
Provera								
Tri-Levlen								
Triphasil								
Tri-Sprintec								
Viagra								
Vivelle-Dot								
Yasmin 28								
Yaz								
Zoladex								

Chapter **24** **Reproductive System**

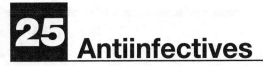

25 Antiinfectives

TERMS AND DEFINITIONS

Select the correct term from the following list and write the corresponding letter in the blank next to the statement.

A. Antibiotic
B. Antimicrobial
C. Bacteria
D. Bactericidal
E. Bacteriostatic
F. ESBLs
G. Gram-negative bacteria
H. Gram-positive bacteria
I. Antibiotic spectrum
J. Inhibit
K. Morphology
L. MRSA
M. Normal flora
N. Nosocomial infection
O. Parasites
P. Pneumonia
Q. PRSP
R. Synthesis
S. Symbiotic
T. Viruses
U. VRE

_____ 1. Unicellular organisms

_____ 2. Organisms that cannot replicate without the necessary components from a host

_____ 3. Bacteria that are unable to keep crystal violet stain when prepared according to Gram-stain procedure

_____ 4. Inflammatory condition of the lungs

_____ 5. Methicillin-resistant *Staphylococcus aureus*

_____ 6. Appearance of an organism, including its shape, size, structure, and Gram staining characteristics

_____ 7. The formation of chemical components in the body systems that comprise cell contents or containers

_____ 8. Agents that prevent the growth of bacteria but do not kill the microbe

_____ 9. Vancomycin-resistant enterococci

_____10. Chemical agents produced by scientists to prevent growth or to kill microorganisms

_____11. Any type of infection a person acquires while hospitalized

_____12. Variety of microbes that a particular antibiotic can treat

_____13. A close working relationship between two species

_____14. Agents that kill bacteria

_____15. Microorganisms that reside harmlessly in the body and do not cause disease, but rather may aid the host organism

_____16. Chemical agents produced by organisms used to treat infection

_____17. To stop or hold back in order to prevent a reaction from taking place

_____18. Extended-spectrum beta-lactamases

_____19. Penicillin-resistant *Streptococcus pneumoniae*

_____20. Bacteria that are able to keep crystal violet stain when prepared using the Gram-stain procedure

_____21. Organisms that require a host for nourishment and reproduction

TRUE OR FALSE

Write T or F next to each statement.

_____ 1. The immune system identifies and neutralizes foreign bodies that have invaded the body.

_____ 2. As patients begin to feel better, they should stop taking their antibiotics.

_____ 3. Penicillin has a more effective bactericidal action on gram-negative bacteria.

_____ 4. Microorganisms have the ability to alter their genetic makeup.

_____ 5. Infections can appear anywhere on or in the body.

_____ 6. Nosocomial infections can be deadly.

_____ 7. Fungi grow only on people who live in moist, warm climates.

_____ 8. Viruses are organisms that live outside their host.

_____ 9. Human immunodeficiency virus (HIV) infection is the precursor to acquired immunodeficiency syndrome (AIDS).

_____ 10. Roundworms can be transferred in undercooked meat.

SYSTEM IDENTIFIER

Label the organs of the immune system and identify the function of each.

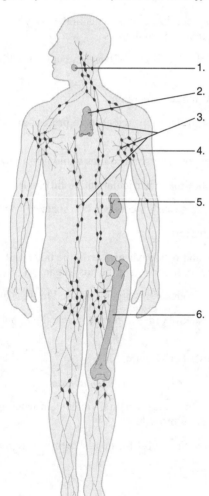

1. _____

2. _____

3. _____

4. _____

5. _____

6. _____

Complete each question by circling the best answer.

1. Which of the following is ***not*** a common type of microorganism?
   A. Bacteria
   B. Fungi
   C. AIDS
   D. Protozoa

2. The main area(s) susceptible to infection is/are the
   A. Genitals
   B. Gastrointestinal (GI) tract
   C. Lungs
   D. All of the above

3. An infection that affects the stomach is
   A. Chlamydia
   B. *Helicobacter pylori*
   C. Tinea
   D. Meningitis

4. Which of the following is ***not*** a common symptom of a respiratory infection?
   A. Wheezing
   B. Coughing
   C. Hiccups
   D. Shortness of breath

5. Tuberculosis (TB) affects which system of the body?
   A. Respiratory system
   B. Cardiovascular system
   C. Urinary system
   D. GI system

6. Individuals at high risk for skin infections are:
   A. Dialysis patients
   B. Diabetic patients
   C. Elderly patients
   D. Pediatric patients

7. Keflex and Suprax are classified as:
   A. Penicillins
   B. Aminoglycosides
   C. Cephalosporins
   D. Antiprotozoans

8. Aminoglycosides can be dangerous because
   A. They come in intravenous (IV) form only
   B. They are given every 4 hours
   C. They are addictive
   D. A narrow range exists between therapeutic and toxic dosages

9. *Candida* infections can occur
   A. In the mouth
   B. In the vagina
   C. Under the nails
   D. All of the above

10. Which of the following is *not* a way that malaria can be transmitted?
    A. Unprotected sex
    B. Infected needles
    C. Mosquitos
    D. Blood

11. What allows a microorganism to avoid the action of antibiotics?
    A. Environment
    B. Resistance
    C. Overuse
    D. None of the above

12. Two compounds combined with amoxicillin and ampicillin, respectively, to strengthen them against microbe resistance are
    A. Hydrochloric acid and sodium chloride
    B. Neosporin and bacitracin
    C. Clavulanic acid and sulbactam
    D. Sodium bicarbonate and Azactam

13. Which of the following organisms is *not* a cause of sexually transmitted diseases (STDs)?
    A. Bacteria
    B. Protozoa
    C. Fungi
    D. Viruses

FILL IN THE BLANK

Answer each question by completing the statement in the space provided.

1. Four antibiotics used to treat *H. pylori* infection of the stomach are _____, _____, _____, and _____.

2. TB is diagnosed by a tuberculin _____ _____ but must be confirmed by a _____ _____ that isolates the bacterium.

3. The two common fungal infections that occur during hospitalization are _____ _____ and _____ _____.

4. The most common eye infection is _____.

5. Antibiotics are often referred to as _____ spectrum and _____ spectrum.

6. The mechanism of action of penicillin is bactericidal toward microbes that are _____ _____.

7. Two main infections in humans caused by a mycobacterium are _____ and _____.

8. The mechanism of action of parenteral aminoglycosides is their ability to _____ to the ribosomes of microorganisms, stopping _____ synthesis.

9. Tinea pedis is commonly known as _____ _____.

10. Viruses require a host's deoxyribonucleic acid (DNA) to _____.

SHORT ANSWER

Write a short response to each question in the space provided. Give examples of drugs from the following drug classes.

1. First-generation penicillin _____

2. Penicillinase-resistant _____

3. Cephalosporins:

   First-generation _____

   Second-generation _____

   Third-generation _____

   Fourt-generation _____

4. Aminoglycoside _____

5. Antiprotozoan _____

6. Antitubercular _____

7. Macrolide _____

MATCHING

Match the following drugs with their classes.

_____ 1. Acyclovir

_____ 2. Mebendazole

_____ 3. Griseofulvin

_____ 4. Keflex

_____ 5. Rifampin

A. Anthelminthic
B. Antibiotic
C. Antituberculin
D. Antifungal
E. Antiviral

Follow the instructions given in each exercise and provide a response.

1. Access the website *www.cdc.gov.*

   A. What are the latest statistics regarding the incidence of HIV/AIDS, TB, and STDs?

   B. Which age group is affected most by each of these diseases?

2. Access the website *http://www.rxlist.com/penicillin-vk-drug.htm.* Read about penicillin and its derivatives and explain their many uses.

REFLECT CRITICALLY

CRITICAL THINKING

Reply to each question based on what you have learned in the chapter.

1. For years, medical researchers have been trying to find the cure for the common cold. Why are common cold viruses so difficult to treat? Why does it seem as if they "keep one step ahead" of the researchers?

2. The immune system can be affected by a hectic lifestyle. What are some contributing factors in your lifestyle that might cause your immune system to function below optimum level?

3. HIV infection is a preventable disease. Make a list of measures you can take to avoid contracting the disease.

4. What is the "invincibility factor" in young adults that makes them take risks while thinking, "It'll never happen to me"?

LAB SCENARIOS

Therapeutic Agents for the Immune System
Objective: To review with the pharmacy technician terms associated with the immune system and review the brand and generic names, indication, contraindications, adverse effects, dosage forms, routes of administration, and recommended daily dosage of medications used to treat disorders of the immune system.

DID YOU KNOW?
- 30.6 million (14%) adults are diagnosed with sinusitis.
- In 2007, there were 13,299 new cases of tuberculosis, 42,995 new cases of salmonella, and 27,444 new cases of Lyme disease.
- In 2008, 28.5% of the children (2 to 17 years), 20% of adults (18 to -49 years), 39% of adults (50 to 64 years) and 67% of adults (65 years and older) received an influenza vaccination.

Lab Activity #25.1: Define the following terms associated with the immune system.

Equipment needed:

- Medical dictionary

- Pencil/pen

Time needed to complete this activity: 30 minutes.

1. AIDS _____

2. Aerobic _____

3. Anaerobic _____

4. Antibodies _____

5. Antiviral resistance _____

6. Bacteria _____

7. Bactericidal _____

8. Bacteriostatic _____

9. HIV _____

10. Immunization _____

11. Immunoglobulins _____

12. Immunosuppressants _____

13. Interferons _____

14. Parasite _____

15. Polyp _____

16. Toxoid vaccine _____

17. Vaccine _____

18. Virostatic _____

19. Virus _____

Lab Activity #25.2: Using a drug reference book, identify the generic name, drug classification, indication, contraindication, adverse effects, dosage forms, routes of administration, and recommended daily dosage of medications used to treat infections.

Equipment needed:

- *Drug Facts & Comparisons* or *Physicians' Desk Reference*
- Pencil/pen

Time needed to complete this activity: 60 minutes.

Brand (Trade) Name	Generic Name	Drug Classification	Indication	List two Contraindications	List five adverse effects	Dosage forms available	Routes of administration	Recommended daily dosage
Amoxil								
Arimidex								
Augmentin								
Avelox								
Avonex								
Bactrim								
Biaxin								
Ceclor								
Ceftin								
Cipro								
Cleocin								
Combivir								
Crixivan								
Doryx								
Enbrel								
Epivir								
Epzicom								
Flagyl								
Keflex								
Kaletra								
Ketek								
Kineret								

Continued

Brand (Trade) Name	Generic Name	Drug Classification	Indication	List two Contraindications	List five adverse effects	Dosage forms available	Routes of administration	Recommended daily dosage
Levaquin								
Minocin								
Neoral								
Norvir								
Rescriptor								
Retrovir								
Septra								
Sumycin								
Suprax								
Sustiva								
Tamiflu								
Trizivir								
Truvada								
Valtrex								
Veetids								
Vibramycin								
Videx								
Vigamox								
Viracept								
Viramune								
Viread								
Zerit								
Zithromax								
Zovirax								

26 Antiinflammatories and Antihistamines

TERMS AND DEFINITIONS

Select the correct term from the following list and write the corresponding letter in the blank next to the statement.

A. Anaphylactic shock
B. Antigen
C. Bradykinins
D. Corticosteroid
E. Debride
F. Histamine
G. Antipyretic
H. Osteoarthritis
I. Rhinitis
J. Steroid
K. Systemic
L. Urticaria
M. Vasodilatation
N. Rheumatoid arthritis
O. Analgesic

_____ 1. Steroid produced by the adrenal cortex

_____ 2. Progressive degenerative and crippling immune disease

_____ 3. A skin eruption of itching wheals

_____ 4. Messenger chemicals produced by the body that help fight inflammation and pain

_____ 5. A substance that interacts with tissues, producing an allergic reaction

_____ 6. A substance that can stimulate an immune response

_____ 7. Pertaining to the whole body rather than to individual body parts

_____ 8. Medication that reduces fever

_____ 9. Drug that relieves pain by reducing the perception of pain

_____10. To remove dead, infected, or damaged tissue

_____11. A severe allergic reaction that causes the blood pressure to decrease rapidly, the heart to go into ventricular tachycardia, and the airways to close; a medical emergency that may cause death immediately

_____12. Inflammation of the lining of the nose; runny nose

_____13. Widening of the blood vessels that allows for increased blood flow

_____14. Chemicals produced by the body that cause inflammation and pain

_____15. Also known as degenerative joint disease

TRUE OR FALSE

Write T or F next to each statement.

_____ 1. Inflammation is a necessary response for the body to heal itself.

_____ 2. Pain is a response that can be measured scientifically.

_____ 3. Acetaminophen is not an antiinflammatory agent.

_____ 4. The first company to market aspirin was St. Joseph's.

_____ 5. Nonsteroidal antiinflammatory drugs (NSAIDs) all work the same; if one brand does not work, neither will another brand.

_____ 6. Steroids have an important role in the maintenance of the body system.

_____ 7. Rheumatoid arthritis is painful and also can cause deformity.

_____ 8. Antihistamines are used to reduce inflammation and irritation.

_____ 9. Histamine can contribute to migraines.

_____10. Anaphylaxis is the most severe case of an allergic reaction but is not deadly.

333

Label the following parts of the skeletal system by putting the correct letter with the corresponding number on the figure.

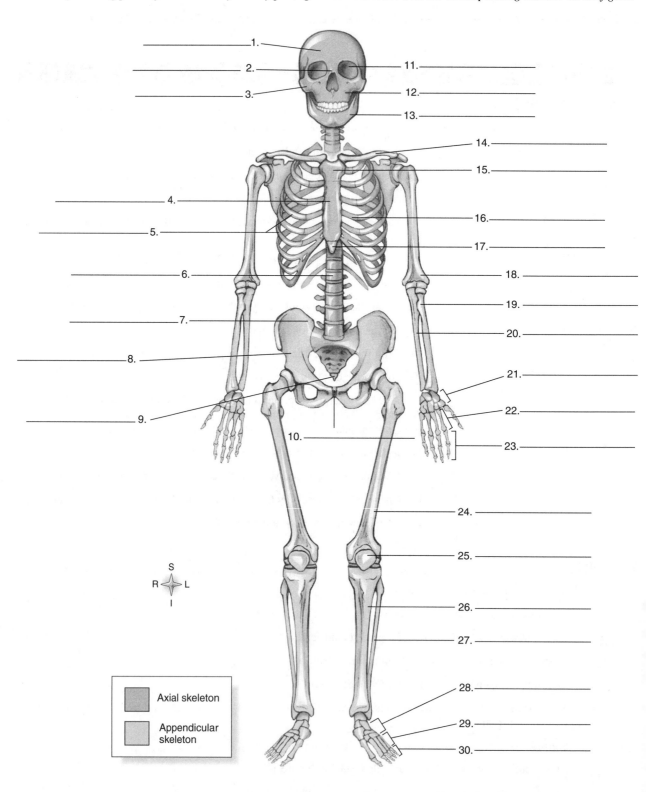

1. _____
2. _____
3. _____
4. _____
5. _____
6. _____
7. _____
8. _____
9. _____
10. _____

11. _____
12. _____
13. _____
14. _____
15. _____
16. _____
17. _____
18. _____
19. _____
20. _____
21. _____
22. _____
23. _____
24. _____
25. _____
26. _____
27. _____
28. _____
29. _____
30. _____

S
R ✦ L
I

Axial skeleton

Appendicular skeleton

Label the following parts of the muscular system by putting the correct letter with the corresponding letter on the figure.

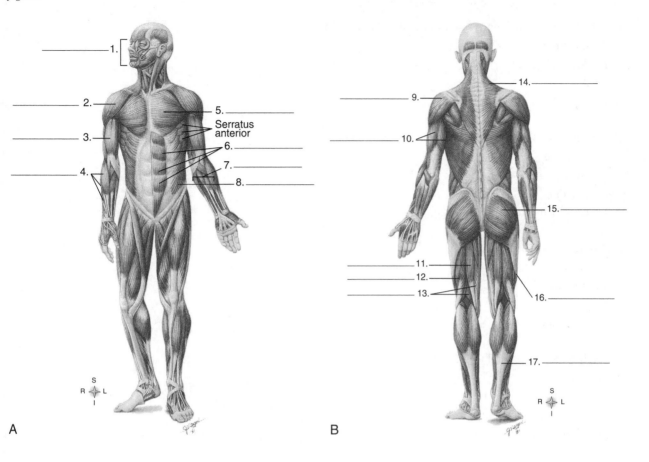

A

B

1.

2.

3.

4.

5.

Serratus anterior

6.

7.

8.

9.

10.

11.

12.

13.

14.

15.

16.

17.

A. Achilles tendon
B. Biceps brachii
C. Biceps femoris
D. Deltoid
E. Extensors of wrists and fingers
F. External abdominal oblique
G. Facial muscles
H. Flexors of wrists and fingers
I. Gluteus maximus
J. Iliotibial tract
K. Pectoralis major
L. Rectus abdominis
M. Semimembranous
N. Semitendinous
O. Patellar tendon abductors of thigh

P. Trapezius
Q. Triceps brachii
R. Patella
S. Phalanges
T. Radius
U. Ribs
V. Sacrum
W. Scapula
X. Sternum
Y. Tarsals
Z. Tibia
AA. Ulna
BB. Vertebral column
CC. Xiphoid process
DD. Zygomatic bone

Complete each question by circling the best answer.

1. Which of the following is **not** a cause of inflammation?
   A. Infection
   B. Advancing age
   C. Allergy
   D. Injury

2. Which of the following is **not** a symptom of inflammation?
   A. Swelling
   B. Heat
   C. Bleeding
   D. Loss of function in the affected area

3. Aspirin is used to treat:
   A. Gout
   B. Inflammation
   C. Fever
   D. All of the above

4. Aspirin therapy is used to prevent:
   A. Stroke
   B. Heart attack
   C. Pulmonary embolism
   D. All of the above

5. Aspirin should not be given to children because its use in that age group has been linked to:
   A. Toxic shock syndrome
   B. Reye's syndrome
   C. Chickenpox
   D. Sudden infant death syndrome (SIDS)

6. Which of the following is true about NSAIDs?
   A. All NSAIDs are available in lesser strengths over the counter (OTC)
   B. They are highly addictive
   C. They reduce fever
   D. They increase inflammation

7. Relafen and Toradol are both:
   A. NSAIDs
   B. Corticosteroids
   C. Antihistamines
   D. Bronchodilators

8. Mast cells are found in tissues of the:
   A. Skin
   B. Gastrointestinal tract
   C. Respiratory tract
   D. All of the above

9. Which of the following is *not* a potential side effect of corticosteroids?
   A. Inflammation
   B. Weight gain
   C. Bruising easily
   D. Moon face

10. Antihistamines work best when taken before:
    A. Eating a meal
    B. An allergic exposure
    C. Going to bed at night
    D. Taking a decongestant

SHORT ANSWER

Write a short response to each question in the space provided.

1. Explain how the enzyme cyclooxygenase affects the body.

   _____

   _____

2. What is Reye's syndrome?

   _____

   _____

3. What three properties do NSAIDs have?

   A. _____

   B. _____

   C. _____

4. What three problems can be caused by the overuse of NSAIDs?

   A. _____

   B. _____

   C. _____

5. Name three common types of medications used to treat asthma.

   A. _____

   B. _____

   C. _____

6. What is the difference between a cyclooxygenase (COX) -1 inhibitor and a COX-2 inhibitor?

_____

_____

_____

_____

_____

_____

MATCHING

Matching I
Match the following trade and generic drug names.

_____ 1. Benadryl   A. Fluticasone
                                    B. Diphenhydramine
_____ 2. Medrol   C. Celecoxib
_____ 3. Flonase   D. Naproxen
                                    E. Methylprednisolone
_____ 4. Celebrex

_____ 5. Anaprox

Matching II
Match the following immune cell responses (see Table 26-1 in text).

_____ 1. Antibodies   A. A globulin found in blood plasma
                                     B. Large cells that secrete cytokines
_____ 2. Leukocytes   C. Large type of leukocyte
_____ 3. Fibrinogen   D. Produced by B lymphocytes
                                     E. White blood cell
_____ 4. Monocyte

_____ 5. Macrophage

RESEARCH ACTIVITY

Follow the instructions given in each exercise and provide a response.

1. Access the website *http://medlineplus.gov.*
   A. Make a list of antihistamines available over the counter.

   B. What are the new asthma inhalers available on the market?

C. Read about insect stings and create a list of treatments.

REFLECT CRITICALLY

CRITICAL THINKING

Reply to each question based on what you have learned in the chapter.

1. You have just been bitten by a fire ant. Knowing that you are severely allergic to these insect bites, what should be your first course of action to prevent anaphylactic shock?

2. TV advertisements can sometimes be deceiving. Picture this: A man is rowing a boat across a lake, and his arms become sore. He comes over to the dock, where his friend awaits him. The rower complains about his arms, and the friend recommends Tylenol for his sore muscles. What is wrong with this picture?

RELATE TO PRACTICE

LAB SCENARIOS

Therapeutic Agents for the Skeletal System

Objective: To review with the pharmacy technician terms associated with the skeletal system and review the brand and generic names, indication, contraindications, adverse effects, dosage forms, routes of administration, and recommended daily dosage of medications used to treat disorders of the skeletal system.

DID YOU KNOW?

- Arthritis affects 51.2 million patients a year.
- Osteoarthritis affects 13.9% of adults aged 25 and older and 33.6% (12.4 million) of those aged 65 and older.
- Women had higher rates of osteoarthritis than men after the age of 50.
- Osteoarthritis accounts for 55% of all arthritis-related hospitalizations.

Lab Activity #26.1: Define the following terms associated with the skeletal system.

Equipment needed:

- Medical dictionary
- Pencil/pen

Time needed to complete this activity: 15 minutes.

1. Gout _____

2. Hyperuricemia _____

3. Osteoarthritis _____

4. Osteoblasts _____

5. Osteoclasts _____

6. Osteopenia _____

7. Osteoporosis _____

8. Paget's disease _____

9. Rheumatoid arthritis _____

Lab Activity #26.2: Using a drug reference book, identify the generic name, drug classification, indication, contraindications, adverse effects, dosage forms, routes of administration, and recommended daily dosage of medications used to treat conditions affecting the skeletal system.

Equipment needed:

- *Drug Facts & Comparisons* or *Physicians' Desk Reference*
- Pencil/pen

Time needed to complete this activity: 20 minutes.

Brand (Trade) Name	Generic Name	Drug Classification	Indication	List Two Contrain-dications	List Five Adverse Effects	Dosage Forms Available	Routes of Administration	Recommended Daily Dosage
Actonel								
Boniva								
Didronel								
Evista								
Fosamax Plus D								
Fosamax								
Miacalcin								
Skelaxin								
Zyloprim								

341

Therapeutic Agents for the Muscular System

Objective: To review with the pharmacy technician terms associated with the muscular system. In addition, to review the brand and generic name, indication, contraindications, adverse effects, dosage forms, routes of administration, and recommended daily dosage of medications used to treat disorders affecting the muscular system.

Lab Activity #26.3: Define the following terms associated with the muscular system.

Equipment needed:

▪ Medical dictionary
▪ Pencil/pen

Time needed to complete this activity: 15 minutes

1. Amyotrophic lateral sclerosis (ALS)

   _____

2. Cerebral palsy

   _____

3. Multiple sclerosis

   _____

4. Muscle strain

   _____

5. Myasthenia gravis

   _____

6. Myositis

   _____

7. Paralysis

   _____

8. Spasticity

   _____

9. Systemic lupus erythematosus

   _____

10. Trigeminal neuralgia

    _____

Lab Activity #26.4: Using a drug reference book, identify the generic name, drug classification, indication, contraindications, adverse effects, dosage forms, routes of administration, and recommended daily dosage of medications used to treat conditions affecting the muscular system.

Equipment needed:

▪ *Drug Facts & Comparisons* or *Physicians' Desk Reference*
▪ Pencil/pen

Time needed to complete this activity: 20 minutes.

342

Brand (Trade) Name	Generic Name	Drug Classification	Indication	List Two Contrain-dications	List Five Adverse Effects	Dosage Forms Available	Routes of Administration	Recommended Daily Dosage
Avonex								
Betaseron								
Dantrium								
Enbrel								
Flexeril								
Humira								
Lioresal								
Parafon Forte								
Prostigmin								
Remicade								
Robaxin								
Soma								
Valium								

Chapter **26** **Antiinflammatories and Antihistamines**

27 Vitamins and Minerals

TERMS AND DEFINITIONS

Select the correct term from the following list and write the corresponding letter in the blank next to the statement.

A. Anemia
B. Avitaminosis
C. Coenzyme
D. Hemoglobin
E. Hypervitaminosis
F. Cofactor
G. Intrinsic factor
H. Trace elements
I. Fat-soluble vitamins
J. Supplement

_____ 1. Compound that activates an enzyme

_____ 2. Vitamins soluble in fat and stored in body fat (A, D, E, and K)

_____ 3. Non-protein chemical compound that is bound to a protein and required for biological activity

_____ 4. Any disease caused by vitamin deficiency or deficiency in metabolic conversion of a vitamin

_____ 5. Iron-containing pigment on red blood cells that carries oxygen to the tissues

_____ 6. Minerals that are required by the body in very small quantities

_____ 7. Condition marked by the presence of an abnormally low number of red blood cells or by a number of dysfunctional red blood cells

_____ 8. A naturally produced protein necessary for the absorption of vitamin B_{12}

_____ 9. Additive to make up for a deficiency such as in vitamins and minerals

_____10. Disorder caused by the intake of too many vitamins; more common with fat-soluble vitamins

TRUE OR FALSE

Write T or F next to each statement.

_____ 1. Vitamins and minerals are necessary for proper growth and development.

_____ 2. Fat-soluble vitamins are stored in the fat cells of the body.

_____ 3. Vitamin supplements are regulated by the Food and Drug Administration (FDA) to ensure ingredient safety.

_____ 4. The FDA regulates the recommended daily intake (RDI) of vitamins and minerals.

_____ 5. All of the B complex vitamins are fat soluble.

_____ 6. Niacin is also known as *nicotine*.

_____ 7. Overcooking vegetables can cause loss of vitamin C.

_____ 8. Minerals are organic substances.

_____ 9. Most of the iron in the body is found in hemoglobin.

_____10. Phospholipids are required for cell membrane formation.

MULTIPLE CHOICE

Complete each question by circling the best answer.

1. Most vitamins and minerals are:
   A. Fat-soluble
   B. Contained in everyday foods
   C. Antioxidants
   D. Prescription only

2. Vitamins A, D, E, and K are all:
   A. Water soluble
   B. Fat soluble
   C. Carbohydrates
   D. Minerals

3. A vitamin D deficiency can cause:
   A. Blindness
   B. Scurvy
   C. Beriberi
   D. Rickets

4. Vitamin K is responsible for:
   A. Blood coagulation factors
   B. Scurvy
   C. Rickets
   D. Lactation

5. All of the B complex vitamins are:
   A. Water soluble
   B. Fat soluble
   C. Carbohydrates
   D. Minerals

6. Which of the following is *not* a major function of thiamine?
   A. Carbohydrate metabolism
   B. Energy production
   C. Red blood cell production
   D. Nervous and cardiovascular system well-being

7. Anemia, dementia, depression, and hair loss can all be caused by a deficiency in:
   A. Vitamin B_3
   B. Vitamin C
   C. Iron
   D. Vitamin B_{12}

8. A vitamin C deficiency can cause:
   A. Beriberi
   B. Hara kari
   C. Rickets
   D. Scurvy

9. Iron deficiency cannot be caused by:
   A. Excessive blood loss
   B. Alcoholism
   C. Erythropoietin
   D. Inadequate intestinal absorption

10. An overdose of calcium can cause:
    A. Kidney stones
    B. Black stools
    C. Scurvy
    D. Osteoporosis

FILL IN THE BLANK

Answer each question by completing the statement in the space provided.

1. Trace elements are agents the body requires to run _____

   _____.

2. The FDA considers all vitamins, minerals, herbs, amino acids, and extracts _____

   _____.

3. Cholecalciferol (vitamin D_3) is produced in the skin in the presence of _____

   _____.

4. Two drugs that interact with vitamin D are _____ and

   _____.

5. The body produces vitamin K by _____ _____ _____

   _____.

6. _____ _____ are vitamins that enable proper cellular functioning of the
   body systems.

7. Three reasons vitamin B_{12} is important for the body are _____

   _____, _____

   _____, and _____

   _____.

8. The main antioxidant vitamins are _____

   _____.

9. Iron is important for the transport of _____ in the blood.

10. The most common type of anemia is _____

   _____.

VITAMIN NAMES

Give the chemical names for the following vitamins.

1. Vitamin A _____

2. Vitamin C _____

3. Vitamin K _____

4. Vitamin B_1 _____

5. Vitamin B_{12} _____

CHEMICAL SYMBOLS

Give the chemical symbols for the following minerals.

1. Calcium _____

2. Chlorine _____

3. Magnesium _____

4. Potassium _____

5. Sodium _____

6. Iron _____

7. Zinc _____

RESEARCH ACTIVITY

Follow the instructions given in each exercise and provide a response.

1. Access the website *http://www.sbaa.org/html/sbaa_facts.html*. Answer the following questions:
   A. What causes spina bifida?

   B. What vitamin is important in the prevention of spina bifida?

2. Visit the local health food store or the vitamin section of your local pharmacy.

   A. Make a list of all the types of calcium supplements available.

   B. What are the active ingredients?

   C. What is the recommended daily dose?

   D. Why is it so important to take vitamin D in conjunction with calcium?

3. Access the website *http://www.merck.com/pubs/mmanual/section1/chapter3/3b.htm*. What are the effects of vitamin A deficiency?

REFLECT CRITICALLY

CRITICAL THINKING

Reply to each question based on what you have learned in the chapter.

1. Have you ever heard of bodybuilders who have vitamin skin odors? Can you really smell like the vitamins you ingest? Explain.

2. Exposure to sunshine activates vitamin D in your body. Does this mean that the more you are exposed to sunshine, the more vitamin D will be activated in your body?

3. Do raw vegetables provide more vitamins than cooked vegetables? Should all vegetables be eaten raw?

4. Most people take vitamins because they feel "run down." Will vitamins really help eliminate that "run down" feeling?

RELATE TO PRACTICE

LAB SCENARIOS

Vitamins and Minerals

Objective: To provide the pharmacy technician the opportunity to demonstrate understanding of vitamins and minerals and their relationship to promoting health.

Vitamins and minerals play an important role in maintaining an individual's health. They are needed for proper growth and development. In most situations, vitamins and minerals are used as supplements to our diet. Many vitamins and minerals can be purchased without a prescription in a variety of retail settings. Often, vitamins and minerals are located close to the pharmacy, resulting in questions to either the pharmacy technician or the pharmacist about their use. Therefore the pharmacy technician needs to be knowledgeable on their use.

Lab Activity #27.1: Using a drug reference book, identify the chemical name, the vitamin's solubility, the recommended daily dosage, indication, adverse effects, and contraindication of each vitamin.

Equipment needed:

- Pencil/pen
- *Drug Facts & Comparison* or *Physicians' Desk Reference for Nutritional Supplements*

Time needed to complete this activity: 15 minutes.

Complete the following table of vitamins.

Vitamin	Chemical Name	Water or Fat Soluble	Prescription (Rx) or Over the Counter(OTC)	Recommended Daily Dosage	Indication	List Two Adverse Effects	List One Contraindication
A							
B1							
B2							
B3							
B5							
B6							
B9							
B12							
C							
D							
E							
K							

Lab Activity #27.2: Using a diagnostic or laboratory test reference, provide the chemical abbreviation of the mineral, its normal range in the blood, and its importance to the human body.

Equipment needed:

- Pencil/pen
- Computer with internet connection
- Diagnostic or laboratory test reference

Time needed to complete this activity: 15 minutes

Complete the following table of minerals.

Mineral	Chemical Abbreviation	Normal Range	Importance of Mineral
Calcium			
Chloride			
Copper			
Iron			
Magnesium			
Manganese			
Phosphorous			
Potassium			
Selenium			
Sodium			
Zinc			

28 Vaccines

TERMS AND DEFINITIONS

Select the correct term from the following list and write the corresponding letter in the blank next to the statement.

A. Acquired immunity
B. Active immunity
C. Antibodies
D. Antigen
E. Attenuated
F. Contagion
G. Globulin
H. Immunity
I. Immunosuppressive agent
J. Lymph node
K. Passive immunity
L. Toxoid
M. Vaccine
N. Virion
O. Virus

_____ 1. Complex molecules made in response to the presence of an antigen that neutralize the effect of the foreign substance

_____ 2. Agents that prevent or lessen the activity of the immune system

_____ 3. Substance that transfers a contagious disease from one individual to another

_____ 4. Immunity acquired by active infection, vaccination, or transfer of products from a donor

_____ 5. Substance that prompts the generation of antibodies and that can produce an immune response

_____ 6. Protein that is insoluble in water

_____ 7. An altered or weakened live vaccine made from the disease organism that the vaccine protects against

_____ 8. Form of acquired immunity in which the body produces its own antibodies against disease-causing antigens

_____ 9. Type of resistance to infection resulting from an immune response from the body in response to an antigen exposure

_____10. Microscopic organism that replicates exclusively inside the host's cell

_____11. Composed of many small oval structures that filter and fight infection and produce lymphocytes and other important immune system cells

_____12. Biologic preparation that improves immunity to a particular disease

_____13. Resistance to a disease that has been acquired through a transfer of antibodies from another person, an animal, or mother to child

_____14. A virus particle

_____15. Type of vaccine in which a toxin has been rendered harmless but still invokes an antigenic response to improve immunity.

TRUE OR FALSE

Write T or F next to each statement.

_____ 1. The lymphatic system is commonly referred to as the *immune system*.

_____ 2. The thymus node is much larger in children than in adults.

_____ 3. Plasma cells make up a major portion of the body's fighting cells.

_____ 4. Through immunizations, society is better protected against disease.

_____ 5. There are two types of immunity, inactive and passive.

_____ 6. With live vaccines, the risk of contracting the full-blown infection from the vaccine is high.

_____ 7. Most vaccines cover either a viral or a bacterial disease that affects humans.

_____ 8. Live virus vaccines must be attenuated before use.

_____ 9. Tetanus vaccine should be given every 6 years for the first 20 years of life.

_____10. Vaccines are available for malaria and fungal infections.

_____11. The main effect of polio is paralysis of the muscles in the legs and the muscles surrounding the lungs.

_____12. If a pregnant mother should contract hepatitis, there is no risk to the fetus.

_____13. Adults receive non-primary vaccinations primarily for travel outside the United States.

_____14. Pregnant women should not receive a measles vaccine because there is a small risk of harm to the fetus.

MULTIPLE CHOICE

Complete each question by circling the best answer.

1. Varicella, MMR, and hepatitis B are all examples of which type of vaccine?
   A. Immune globulin
   B. Antivenins
   C. Viral
   D. Toxoids

2. The larger nodes of the lymphatic system are:
   A. Thymus
   B. Tonsils
   C. Spleen
   D. All of the above

3. The primary function of the thymus is to produce:
   A. Lymphocytes
   B. Antivenins
   C. Immune globulins
   D. Interferon

4. The function of the spleen is to:
   A. Destroy old blood cells
   B. Destroy bacteria and foreign bodies
   C. A and B
   D. None of the above

354

5. Lymphocytes produce:
   A. B cells
   B. T cells
   C. More lymphocytes
   D. Plasma cells

6. A weakened form of antigen vaccine is given for:
   A. Whooping cough
   B. Tetanus
   C. Polio
   D. All of the above

7. Which of the following is *not* a person at high risk for catching and succumbing to disease?
   A. Chemotherapy patient
   B. Adolescent patient
   C. Transplant patient
   D. Acquired immunodeficiency syndrome (AIDS) patient

8. Which type of immunity protects from an outside source such as an immunization vaccine?
   A. Active immunity
   B. Passive immunity
   C. Both A and B
   D. Neither A nor B

9. In the United States, children cannot register for school unless they:
   A. Have obtained and filed appropriate religious exemptions
   B. Have proof of immunizations
   C. Have obtained and filed appropriate medical exemptions
   D. All of the above

10. One vaccine that protects against meningitis is called:
    A. Havrix
    B. Varivax
    C. Pneumonococcal polysaccharide vaccine
    D. Cytomegalovirus immune globulin

FILL IN THE BLANK

Answer each question by completing the statement in the space provided.

1. When first contact is made with a foreign body (antigen), _____ are formed.

2. _____ and _____ recommend the course of vaccinations for children.

3. _____ _____ _____ occurs when the body is exposed to a disease and actively produces antibodies.

4. Some vaccines are referred to as _____, which are inactivated _____ toxins.

5. The hepatitis B virus is transmitted through _____ and _____

   _____.

6. Another name for *pertussis* is _____ _____; another name for *tetanus* is

_____.

7. Mumps affect the _____ glands of the body.

8. The virus that causes chickenpox can also cause _____.

9. Two medications used for shingles are _____ and _____.

10. Immune globulins are attained from a _____ or _____ donor.

11. The only persons authorized to receive the anthrax vaccine are those in the _____.

MATCHING

Match the following types of vaccines with their sources.

_____ 1. Rabies

_____ 2. Tetanus

_____ 3. Hepatitis B

_____ 4. Etanercept

_____ 5. Cyclosporine

A. Viral
B. Biologic response modifier
C. Toxoid
D. Immunosuppressive
E. Antitoxin

RESEARCH ACTIVITY

Follow the instructions given in each exercise and provide a response.

1. Access the website *www.cdc.gov.*
   A. What was the latest released?

   B. How many strains of the hepatitis virus are currently known? How many vaccines are available and to what strain(s)?

2. Access the website *http://www.medformation.com/mf/stayhealthy.nsf/page/immunizechild.* Print the pediatric immunization schedule. How many vaccinations are required for children aged 0 to 4 years?

3. Access the website *http://www.cdc.gov/nip/recs/adult-schedule.pdf.* Print the adult immunization schedule. How many vaccinations are required for adults?

CRITICAL THINKING

Reply to each question based on what you have learned in the chapter.

1. Human immunodeficiency virus (HIV) infection can be a devastating disease. What type of lymphocyte is most important for patients with HIV infection? Why?

2. In the United States, sanitization and hygiene are stressed, yet people still frequently become ill. Does constant sanitization bring about a healthier immune system or does it weaken it?

3. Botulinum toxin (example: Botox) is the latest product being used to "reduce or eliminate wrinkles." Can repeated Botox injections harm the recipients or cause them to build up a resistance to the toxin?

4. The World Health Organization (WHO) has been working tirelessly to eradicate infectious diseases throughout the world, with much success. What would happen to the planet's population if all infectious diseases were eradicated and vaccinations were not needed?

RELATE TO PRACTICE

LAB SCENARIOS

Vaccines

Objective: To introduce the pharmacy technician to the use of vaccines in the practice of pharmacy.

Lab Activity #28.1: Researching seasonal influenza. Using the Centers for Disease Control and Prevention website *(www.cdc.gov/flu/)*, answer the following questions regarding seasonal influenza.

Equipment needed:

- Pencil/pen
- Computer with internet connection
- Paper

Time needed to complete this activity: 45 minutes.

1. Who should be vaccinated for seasonal influenza?

_____

_____

_____

_____

2. What are some of the symptoms of seasonal influenza?

_____

_____

_____

_____

_____

3. Who is at risk for contacting the flu?

_____

_____

_____

_____

4. How does the flu spread from individual to individual?

_____

_____

_____

_____

_____

5. What are three ways to protect one from getting seasonal influenza?

_____

_____

_____

_____

_____

6. What is the composition of the current flu vaccine?

_____

_____

_____

_____

7. At what temperature should the flu vaccine be stored?

_____

_____

_____

_____

8. In which month do we experience the greatest number of cases of the flu?

_____

9. What antiviral medications may be used in the treatment of seasonal influenza?

_____

10. Complete the following table.

Trade Name	Manufacturer	Presentation	Mercury Content	Age Group	Number of Doses	Route of Administration
Fluzone		0.25 ml prefilled syringe				
		0.5 ml prefilled syringe				
		0.5 ml vial				
		5.0 ml multi-dose vial				
Fluvirin		5.0 ml multi-dose vial				
		0.5 ml prefilled syringe				
Agriflu		0.5 ml prefilled syringe				
Fluarix		0.5 ml prefilled syringe				
FluLaval		5.0 ml multi-dose vial				
Afluria		0.5 ml prefilled syringe				
Fluzone High-Dose		0.5 ml prefilled syringe				
FluMist		0.2 ml sprayer				

Objective: Obtain information on immunization training requirements within your state.

Lab Activity #28.2: Using the internet to research information on the criteria to immunize customers (patients) in your state and complete the following table.

Equipment needed:

- Computer with Internet connection
- Pencil/pen

Time needed to complete this activity: 30 minutes

What is the name of your state?	
Who may immunize pharmacy customers?	
What immunizations may they perform?	
Describe the training required to be able to immunize a customer?	
Does an individual require clinical training before being permitted to immunize patients?	
Does an individual need to register with a regulatory agency in the state? If yes, which agency?	
Does an individual need to be licensed to immunize customers?	
What does it cost to be able to immunize customers?	
Does an individual need continuing education for the renewal of their registration or license? If so, how many CEUs are needed annually?	

Objective: Retail pharmacy visit.

Lab Activity #28.3: Visit a retail pharmacy that offers flu shots or other immunizations to their customers. Ask for a copy of the paperwork that the patient must fill out before receiving an immunization.

Equipment Needed:

- None

Time needed to complete this activity: 15 minutes

1. Compare and contrast the information found on the sheet with other members of your class. What is the same? What is different?

_____

_____

_____

_____

_____

2. Does medical or prescription drug coverage pay for the immunization?

_____

_____

_____

_____

Lab Activity #28.4: Use the Centers for Disease Control and Prevention (CDC) website (www. cdc.gov/vaccines) to identify the generic name, indication, contraindication, adverse effect, and the routes of administration of the vaccines listed in the following tables.

Equipment needed:

- Computer with Internet connection
- Pencil/pen

Time needed to complete this activity: 45 minutes.

Brand (Trade) Name	Generic Name	Indication	List Two Contraindications	List Five Adverse Effects	Routes of Administration
Adacel					
BioThrax					
Boostrix					
Cervarix					
Daptacel					
Dryvax					
Engerix-B					
Gardasil					
Havrix					
Imovax Rabies					
Infanrix					
IPOL					
Ixiaro					
JE-Vax					
Kinrix					
Menactra					
Menomune					

Brand (Trade) Name	Generic Name	Indication	List Two Contraindications	List Five Adverse Effects	Routes of Administration
Menveo					
M-M-R II					
Pediarix					
Pentacel					
Pneumovax 23					
Prevnar					
ProQuad					
Recombivax HB					
Rotarix					
Tripedia					
Twinrix					
Varivax					
Vivotif					
YF-Vax					
Zostavax					

29 Oncology Agents

TERMS AND DEFINITIONS

Select the correct term from the following list and write the corresponding letter in the blank next to the statement.

A. Antineoplastic
B. Benign
C. Biopsy
D. Cancer
E. Carcinogen
F. Chemotherapy
G. Deoxyribonucleic acid (DNA)
H. Invasive
I. Oncologist
J. Lymphoma
K. Malignant
L. Melanoma
M. Metastasis
N. Mitosis
O. Mortality
P. Mutation
Q. Neoplasm
R. Oncogene
S. Remission
T. Stage

_____ 1. Gene that when mutated, can help turn a normal cell into a cancerous one

_____ 2. Procedure in which a piece of tissue is removed for examination and diagnosis

_____ 3. Being susceptible to death

_____ 4. Treatment of a disease with toxic chemicals to slow the disease process

_____ 5. Malignant neoplasm of the pigmented cells of skin; may metastasize to other organs

_____ 6. Specialist in the area of cancer and cancer treatment

_____ 7. General term used to describe malignant neoplasms or tumors

_____ 8. An abnormal tissue growth

_____ 9. Tendency for a tumor or mass to move into tissues or organs in proximity

_____ 10. Tumor or growth that is not life-threatening

_____ 11. Double helix structure containing the complex nucleic acids sequences that are bases for genetic continuance

_____ 12. Movement or spread of cancerous cells through the body to organs in distant areas

_____ 13. Span of time during which a disease is not spreading/progressing; it may even be diminished or cured

_____ 14. Cellular reproduction that creates two identical daughter cells from a parent cell's DNA

_____ 15. Substance or chemical that can increase the risk of developing cancer

_____ 16. An invasive, destructive pattern of rapid, abnormal cell growth that is often fatal

_____ 17. Unexpected change in molecular structure within DNA causes permanent change

_____ 18. Describes the extent of cancer within the body and its spread to other areas

_____ 19. Medication used in treatment of abnormal cells

_____ 20. A term used to describe a malignant disorder of lymphoid tissue

TRUE OR FALSE

Write T or F next to each statement.

_____ 1. If a person has cancer, it certainly means death.

_____ 2. Cancer can strike any area of the body.

_____ 3. Benign tumors are cancerous.

_____ 4. Cancer can be caused by environmental contaminants.

_____ 5. If some types of cancer are diagnosed in the early stages, they may be surgically removed.

_____ 6. Fewer than 100 known cancers plague the human body.

_____ 7. Kaposi's sarcoma is a rare type of cancer that affects the skin.

_____ 8. The risk of cancer declines as a person ages beyond 65 years.

_____ 9. Surgery is frequently used in the diagnosis and treatment of cancer.

_____10. Many chemotherapeutic agents destroy healthy cells along with cancer cells.

MULTIPLE CHOICE

Complete each question by circling the best answer.

1. Which of the following is *not* a form that can turn into a malignant or cancerous tumor?
   A. Pimples
   B. Moles
   C. Warts
   D. Lesions

2. Which of the following is *not* a type of cancer?
   A. Carcinoma
   B. Leukemia
   C. Lymphoma
   D. Bulimia

3. Some types of cancer-causing agents include:
   A. Radioactive materials
   B. Coal
   C. Dyes
   D. All of the above

4. Which of the following is *not* a means by which cancers can be identified and treated?
   A. Magnetic resonance imaging (MRI)
   B. Electrocardiogram (EKG)
   C. Sonogram
   D. Biopsy

5. Breast and prostate cancers are being cured more often as a result of:
   A. Examinations/early detection
   B. Vaccines
   C. A and B
   D. None of the above

364

6. Leukemia arises in the:
   A. Bone marrow
   B. Lymphatic system
   C. A and B
   D. None of the above

7. Treatments for cancer include all of the following *except:*
   A. Surgery
   B. Radiation
   C. Vitamins
   D. Chemotherapy

8. Cytarabine, fluorouracil, and methotrexate are:
   A. Mitotic inhibitors
   B. Antibiotics
   C. Alkylating agents
   D. Antimetabolites

9. Nitrogen mustards were first used in:
   A. The Vietnam War
   B. The Korean War
   C. World War I
   D. World War II

10. A nuclear pharmacy technician must wear a:
    A. Badge stating that the person is a nuclear technician
    B. Radioactive meter
    C. Lead apron
    D. All of the above

FILL IN THE BLANK

Answer each question by completing the statement in the space provided.

1. _____ lymphoma is a common cancer of the lymphatic cell located in the lymph node.

2. Most treatments for cancer include more than one _____ and may be followed up with or preceded by _____ therapy.

3. Radiation is classified by the _____ of the rays. Alpha and beta rays are used to treat _____ lesions, gamma rays are used to treat _____ lesions.

4. Antimetabolites are often used in the treatment of _____.

5. Side effects of antineoplastic antibiotics used in cancer treatment include: _____, _____, _____, _____ _____, and _____ _____.

6. Vinblastine and vincristine are _____ derived from plants.

7. Two major types of alkylating agents are _____ _____ and _____.

365

8. _____ are agents that cross blood-brain barrier and can be used to treat

   _____ cancer.

9. Two main biologic response modifiers used to treat side effects of chemotherapy are _____ and

   _____.

10. Agents used in nuclear pharmacy are called _____.

MATCHING

Matching I

Match the following drugs with their classification.

_____ 1. Bleomycin

_____ 2. Cyclophosphamide

_____ 3. Methotrexate

_____ 4. Vinblastine

_____ 5. Topotecan

A. Alkylating agent
B. Topoisomerase inhibitor
C. Antimitotic
D. Antibiotic
E. Antimetabolite

Matching II

Match the following drugs with their indications.

_____ 1. Vinorelbine

_____ 2. Paclitaxel

_____ 3. Cytarabine

_____ 4. Dactinomycin

_____ 5. Ifosfamide

A. Myelocytic leukemia
B. Testicular cancer
C. Lung cancer
D. Ovarian/breast cancer
E. Wilms' tumor

RESEARCH ACTIVITY

Follow the instructions given in each exercise and provide a response.

1. Access the website *www.cancerguide.org*. Take the tour of the website to see what kind of information is offered. Summarize what you have learned.

2. Access the website *www.cancer.gov*. Choose the section Statistics. Choose two types of cancers and list the latest statistics on them.

3. Access the website *http://www.cancerquest.org/index.cfm?page=183*. List the various types of cancer treatments discussed.

4. Can a known poison be used to treat cancer?

REFLECT CRITICALLY

CRITICAL THINKING

Reply to each question based on what you have learned in the chapter.

1. A woman poses this question to her doctor: "My grandmother, aunt, and cousin all died of breast cancer. Does it mean that I will get cancer, too?"
   A. Is cancer hereditary?

   B. Should the woman be thinking about a mastectomy, even if she does not currently have cancer?

2. Many scientists claim that the cure for cancer lies in the plants of the world's great forests. These forests are disappearing as a result of the growth in the world's population and the use of land for mining or to grow food. Should governments get involved in plant-targeted cancer research? What can be done to foster research in this area?

3. Tobacco is a known carcinogen, yet people still use it. What would you use to illustrate the devastating effects of tobacco on the respiratory system?

LAB SCENARIOS

Therapeutic Agents for the Oncology

Objective: To review the brand and generic names, indication, contraindications, adverse effects, dosage forms, routes of administration, and recommended daily dosage of medications used to treat cancer.

DID YOU KNOW?

- 17.9 million (7.9%) adults have been diagnosed with cancer.
- Cancer ranks second as a leading cause of death.
- In 2006, there were 40,821 deaths attributed to breast cancer.
- In 2000, there were 8,100 (7.7%) current patients with prostate cancer as the primary diagnosis.

Lab Activity #29.1: Using a drug reference book, identify the generic name, drug classification, indication, contraindication, adverse effects, dosage forms, routes of administration, and recommended daily dosage of medications used to treat cancer and related disorders.

Equipment needed:

- *Drug Facts & Comparisons* or *Physicians' Desk Reference*
- Pencil/pen

Time needed to complete this activity: 30 minutes.

Brand (Trade) Name	Generic Name	Drug Classification	Indication	List Two Contraindications	List Five Adverse Effects	Dosage Forms Available	Routes of Administration	Recommended Daily Dosage
Adriamycin								
Alkeran								
Arimidex								
BiCNU								
CCNU								
CellCept								
Cerubidine								
Cosmegen								
Cytoxan								
Fludara								
Fuzeon								
Gemzar								
Hycamtin								
Hydrea								
Iressa								
Leukeran								
Matulane								
Megace								

Continued

Brand (Trade) Name	Generic Name	Drug Classification	Indication	List Two Contraindications	List Five Adverse Effects	Dosage Forms Available	Routes of Administration	Recommended Daily Dosage
Methotrexate								
Myleran								
Navelbine								
Nipent								
Nolvadex								
Oncovin								
Paraplatin								
Platinol AQ								
Purinethol								
Purinethol								
Taxol								
Taxotere								
Velban								
VePesid								
Vumon								
Xeloda								
Zanosar								
Zoladex								

30 Microbiology

TERMS AND DEFINITIONS

Select the correct term from the following list and write the corresponding letter in the blank next to the statement.

A. Aerobic
B. Anaerobic
C. Binary fission
D. Biology
E. Catalyst
F. Enzyme
G. Facultative anaerobe
H. Heterotrophic
I. Microbial
J. Microbiology
K. Morphology
L. Peptidoglycan
M. Species
N. Taxonomy
O. Vector
P. Virology
Q. Virus

_____ 1. Entity by which infections are transferred; entity of transference does not have disease and does not need to be living

_____ 2. The method of non-sexual reproduction by which a single cell divides into two separate cells

_____ 3. Polymer substance that comprises bacterial cell walls

_____ 4. Protein that speeds up a reaction by reducing the amount of energy required to initiate a reaction

_____ 5. Refers to microorganisms not visible without a microscope

_____ 6. Organisms that need oxygen to survive

_____ 7. Microscopic organism that replicates exclusively inside the host's cell

_____ 8. Latin origin meaning "kind"; in biology the basic rank in taxonomic classification

_____ 9. Molecule that allows chemical reactions to take place rapidly but is not altered in the reaction

_____10. Requiring complex carbon and nitrogen for metabolic synthesis

_____11. Organisms that live in the absence of oxygen

_____12. Study of microscopic organisms

_____13. Study of viruses

_____14. Microorganism that can live with or without oxygen

_____15. Hierarchical structure for the nomenclature and classification of organisms

_____16. Study of life

_____17. Study of the features of organisms without studying the function of organisms

TRUE OR FALSE

Write T or F next to each statement.

_____ 1. Viruses are smaller than bacteria.

_____ 2. Louis Pasteur's lifetime was called the *golden age of biology*.

_____ 3. The study of naming and classifying organisms is called *taxidermy*.

_____ 4. Viruses are not included in the traditional taxonomic kingdoms.

_____ 5. Plants acquire energy differently from animals.

_____ 6. Many diseases are transmitted easily by plants.

_____ 7. Animal cells get their energy from food rather than from sunlight.

_____ 8. Vectors are the carriers of organisms or genetic materials to a host.

_____ 9. Algae do not need light to survive.

_____10. Humans are more susceptible to fungal infections than plants are.

MULTIPLE CHOICE

Complete each question by circling the best answer.

1. The study of microbiology includes all of the following:
   A. Bacteria
   B. Fungi
   C. Protists
   D. All of the above

2. The first microscope was invented by:
   A. Gregory Hacker
   B. Herbert Ritchie
   C. Robert Hooke
   D. Steven Martin

3. It was believed that flies came from:
   A. Manure
   B. Decaying corpses
   C. Snakes
   D. All of the above

4. Louis Pasteur proved that:
   A. Unseen microorganisms exist in the air
   B. Deoxyribonucleic acid (DNA) is a genetic material
   C. Cleaning the hands between surgeries reduces the spread of infection
   D. All of the above

5. The plant kingdom includes all of the following *except:*
   A. Mosses
   B. Viruses
   C. Ferns
   D. Conifers

372

6. Plants have chloroplasts, which are used to:
   A. Convert sunlight to energy
   B. Convert sunlight to fragrance
   C. Convert energy to fragrance
   D. Convert fragrance to energy

7. Which of the following is *not* a way people benefit from plants?
   A. Food
   B. Clothing
   C. Touch
   D. Building materials

8. Which of the following is *not* an example of a complex animal organism?
   A. Frog
   B. Sponge
   C. Kangaroo
   D. Spider

9. Dysentery is spread by transfer from:
   A. Penis to cervix
   B. Cervix to penis
   C. Foot to mouth
   D. Feces to mouth

10. Conditions that may be caused by a fungus are:
    A. Athlete's foot
    B. Sepsis
    C. Vaginal infections
    D. All of the above

FILL IN THE BLANK

Answer each question by completing the statement in the space provided.

1. One difference between eukaryotes and prokaryotes is that eukaryotes have a _____ and prokaryotes do not.

2. Digoxin is taken from the _____ plant and is used to treat _____ conditions.

3. *Trichomonas vaginalis* is a _____ that causes infection in the male

   _____ _____ and in the _____ of

   females.

4. The fungi kingdom is divided into _____ fungi and _____

   _____.

5. _____ are responsible for decomposing plant organisms.

6. *Candida albicans* is part of _____ _____ in the mouth and genitourinary tract of humans.

7. Penicillin destroys _____ by interacting with _____ present in the cell walls of bacteria.

8. _____ destroy bacteria by breaking down their cell walls.

9. The enzyme that renders the penicillins useless against bacteria is _____.

10. Narrow-spectrum antibiotics primarily act against _____ _____

microbes, and broad-spectrum antibiotics include coverage against _____

_____ microbes.

SHORT ANSWER

Write a short response to each question in the space provided.

1. How are viruses classified?

_____

_____

_____

2. How do viruses survive?

_____

_____

_____

3. How are viruses identified?

_____

_____

_____

4. How does the drug zidovudine work?

_____

_____

_____

MATCHING

Match the microbe with the correct disease or condition.

_____ 1. Protozoan

_____ 2. Bacterium

_____ 3. Virus

_____ 4. Helminth

_____ 5. Fungus

A. Human immunodeficiency virus (HIV)
B. Roundworms
C. Malaria
D. Ringworm
E. Meningitis

RESEARCH ACTIVITY

Follow the instructions given in each exercise and provide a response.

1. Access the website *http://co.howard.in.us/health/insect.htm* and learn about vectors of disease. Summarize what you have learned.

2. Access the website *http://poisonivy.aesir.com/* and learn facts about poison ivy and poison oak. Summarize what you have learned.

REFLECT CRITICALLY

CRITICAL THINKING

Reply to each question based on what you have learned in the chapter.

1. If you had the chance to do an educational presentation on HIV/AIDS, what five things would you stress most in your presentation?

2. Many companies market antibacterial soaps, cleansers, and so forth. What would be the result of overuse of these products?

3. Handwashing is one of the most important tools for universal precautions and for preventing the spread of germs. What tool can you use to convince children and adults to teach about the importance of handwashing?

RELATE TO PRACTICE

LAB SCENARIOS

Gram Stain Lab Procedure

Objective: To provide a step-by-step procedure for performing a Gram stain.

Lab Activity #30.1 Gain confidence in viewing organisms through a microscope and understand the purpose of the staining process by following the procedure below.

Equipment needed:

- Glass slide
- Small tongs or large tweezers
- Marker
- Square plastic slide cover
- Toothpicks
- Iodine dropper bottle
- Violet dropper bottle
- Water dropper bottle
- Long lighter
- Microscope

Time needed to complete this activity: 60 minutes

Step-by-Step Procedure

1. Draw a circle on the underside of the glass side (the top side will hold the sample).

2. Lightly scrape the inside of your cheek with the toothpick.

3. Scrape the toothpick onto the top of the glass slide (the side not marked with the circle).

4. Use tongs or tweezers to hold the slide at the edge. Wave the lighter back and forth quickly three times under the slide; this sets the cells onto the slide.

5. Over a sink or pan, apply the solutions.

6. Place one drop of iodine. Wait 1 minute, and then rinse with water.

7. Place one drop of violet. Wait 1 minute, and then rinse with water.

8. Place the plastic slide cover over the sample and view the sample under the microscope.

9. First, view at 10 degrees; draw what you see.

10. Then, view at 40 degrees; draw what you see.

Safety Tips

1. When using anything glass, always handle the article extremely carefully to avoid breaking it or injuring yourself with an intact or a broken item.

2. If glass breaks, clean up and dispose of the item according to institutional procedures.

3. Use caution when scraping the inside of your cheek with the toothpick. Do not poke your cheek because this can cause injury.

4. Be extremely careful when using an open flame; do not leave it unattended.

5. Always wipe the eyepieces of the microscope with alcohol before and after using the instrument to reduce the chance of spreading infection.

31 Chemistry

TERMS AND DEFINITIONS

Select the correct term from the following list and write the corresponding letter in the blank next to the statement.

A. Amino acids
B. Anabolism
C. Atom
D. Catabolism
E. Covalent bond
F. Electron
G. Enzyme
H. Ion
I. Ionic bond
J. Macro
K. Metabolism
L. Micro
M. Mole
N. Molecule
O. Neutron
P. Nucleic acid
Q. Atomic orbit
R. Proton

_____ 1. Smallest unit of an element, composed of a nucleus surrounded by electrons

_____ 2. Sharing of electrons between two atoms

_____ 3. Transfer of electrons between two atoms

_____ 4. Subset of an atom that does not contain a charge

_____ 5. Subatomic particle of an atom that holds a positive charge

_____ 6. Bases contained within deoxyribonucleic acid (DNA)

_____ 7. Large

_____ 8. Protein that speeds up a reaction by reducing the amount of energy required to initiate a reaction

_____ 9. To break down; the destruction phase of metabolism

_____10. Small

_____11. Rotational path of electrons around the nucleus

_____12. Avogadro's number; 6.02×10^{23} atoms, molecules, or ions

_____13. Smallest subset of an atom that contains a negative charge

_____14. An atom or group of atoms with a leftover unbalanced charge

_____15. Macromolecules that make up proteins

_____16. Physical and chemical change that takes place within an organism

_____17. Smallest particle of a compound

_____18. To build up; the construction phase of metabolism

TRUE OR FALSE

Write T or F next to each statement.

_____ 1. Chemistry has little to do with the health care field.

_____ 2. The nucleus of an atom is very small.

_____ 3. Enzymatic reactions can speed up a reaction pathway.

_____ 4. Chemical reactions make life happen.

_____ 5. The human body needs nutrients on a monthly basis.

_____ 6. Aminoglycosides can build up in the blood and certain body tissues.

_____ 7. To ensure sterility, a new total parenteral nutrition (TPN) must be hung every week.

_____ 8. Each TPN is tailor-made to the patient's specific needs.

_____ 9. Copper is a metal the body uses in minute amounts.

_____10. Iodine is needed for proper functioning of the kidney.

MULTIPLE CHOICE

Complete each question by circling the best answer.

1. Each atom has the same number of protons and electrons; therefore it is:
   A. Positive
   B. Negative
   C. Neutral
   D. None of the above

2. Organic chemistry is the study of:
   A. Substances that contain carbon
   B. Substances that contain dioxide
   C. Substances that contain oxygen
   D. All of the above

3. Enzymes are composed of elements that can cause:
   A. A reaction
   B. A faster reaction
   C. A reaction to stop
   D. All of the above

4. Which patient will *not* require a TPN?
   A. A patient who cannot eat food for prolonged periods
   B. A patient with bowel obstruction
   C. A patient healing from stomach surgery
   D. None of the above

5. Zinc is needed in:
   A. Large amounts
   B. Very minute amounts
   C. All vitamin preparations
   D. None of the above

6. When amino acids join together, they cause:
   A. Dehydration
   B. Proteins to be made
   C. Nausea and vomiting
   D. Diarrhea

7. Metabolism is necessary for the control of:
   A. Hormones
   B. Protein synthesis
   C. pH, fat, and glucose levels
   D. All of the above

8. Neutrons are:
   A. Positively charged
   B. Negatively charged
   C. Not charged
   D. A and B

9. Which of the following are made by joining two or more atoms?
   A. Carbohydrates
   B. Lipids
   C. Proteins
   D. All of the above

10. The human body is composed of _____ of molecules:
   A. Thousands
   B. Millions
   C. Hundreds
   D. Billions

SHORT ANSWER

Write a short response to each question in the space provided.

1. How is the salt NaCl used in the hospital?

   _____

   _____

2. Inorganic chemistry is the study of:

   _____

   _____

3. Organic chemistry is the study of:

   _____

   _____

4. What is the purpose of lab tests as they relate to monitoring medications or nutrition?

   _____

   _____

5. What are the main ingredients of a hyperal (TPN) bag?

   _____

   _____

6. What other ingredients are contained in the TPN?

   _____

   _____

7. Where is most phosphorus found in the body, and what enzyme does it help to make?

_____

_____

8. What is the range of the pH scale, and what is the normal pH range of the blood?

_____

_____

9. How many main amino acids are there and for what are they used?

_____

_____

FILL IN THE BLANK

Answer each question by completing the statement in the space provided.

1. The two types of bonding between atoms are _____ and _____.

2. The _____ _____ of elements has all the known elements strategically placed according to their properties.

3. The metal _____ by itself is highly reactive and would explode if it came in contact with oxygen.

4. Hydrogen peroxide is used as an _____ in households.

5. The human body is able to produce energy and perform other functions quickly because of _____.

CHEMICAL COMPOUNDS

Give the formula for the following chemical compounds.

1. Water _____

2. Ferrous sulfate _____

3. Sodium chloride _____

4. Potassium chloride _____

5. Hydrochloric acid _____

6. Sodium bicarbonate _____

RESEARCH ACTIVITY

Follow the instructions given in each exercise and provide a response.

1. Access the website *http://www.nyu.edu/pages/mathmol/library/drugs/index.html*. Look at the chemical structures for the various drugs. Summarize what you have learned.

REFLECT CRITICALLY

CRITICAL THINKING

Reply to each question based on what you have learned in the chapter.

1. You went out on Friday night for pizza and a movie with friends. During the course of the evening, in addition to pizza, you ate popcorn and candy and drank soda. By the end of the night you were extremely thirsty. What chemical compounds in the pizza, popcorn, and soda contributed to your thirst?

2. Is ammonia (NH_4), a byproduct produced in the body, the same type of ammonia you can buy in the grocery store?

3. If you were to market a drink that contained all the chemicals the body needs, what would your ingredients be?